The Nursing Associate

The Nursing Associate

Stepping into Practice

Edited by

Annabel Coulson
University Hospitals of Leicester NHS Trust
Leicester, UK

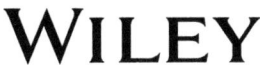

This edition first published 2025
© 2025 by John Wiley & Sons Ltd

The right of Annabel Coulson to be identified as the author of the editorial material in this work has been asserted in accordance with law.

Registered Office(s)
John Wiley & Sons, Inc., 111 River Street, Hoboken, NJ 07030, USA
John Wiley & Sons Ltd, New Era House, 8 Oldlands Way, Bognor Regis, West Sussex, PO22 9NQ, UK

For details of our global editorial offices, customer services, and more information about Wiley products visit us at www.wiley.com.

The manufacturer's authorized representative according to the EU General Product Safety Regulation is Wiley-VCH GmbH, Boschstr. 12, 69469 Weinheim, Germany, e-mail: Product_Safety@wiley.com. Wiley also publishes its books in a variety of electronic formats and by print-on-demand. Some content that appears in standard print versions of this book may not be available in other formats.

Library of Congress Cataloging-in-Publication Data Applied for:

Paperback ISBN: 9781119698562

Cover Design: Wiley
Cover Image: © NAMPIX/Adobe Stock Photos

Set in 11.5/13.5 STIXTwoText by Straive, Pondicherry, India
Printed and bound by CPI Group (UK) Ltd, Croydon, CR0 4YY

C9781119698562_150325

Contents

Leigh-Ann Cowell

  Introduction. 51

  Aims of This Chapter 51

  Related NMC Standards. 52

  What Is Person-centred Care? 52

  Nursing Theories and Models 55

  Popular Nursing Models 56

    Orem (1980) 56

    Peplau's Theory of Nursing (1991) 56

    Roper, Logan and Tierney (2000) 57

    Recovery Star 57

  The Nursing Process. 58

  Patient and Family-centred Care 59

  Person-centred Care at End of Life 61

  Supporting Person-centred Care with Cultural Competence 62

    Cultural Awareness 63

    Cultural Knowledge. 63

    Cultural Skill 63

    Cultural Encounters. 63

    Cultural Desire 63

  Chapter Summary. 64

  References 64

  Further Reading 65

5 Effective Communication for the Nursing Associate 67
Michelle Richardson

  Introduction. 67

  Aims of This Chapter 67

  Related to NMC Standards 67

  The Importance of 'Good' Communication 68

  Underpinning Theories 68

  Understanding Ourselves and How We Develop Our Own
  Communication. 69

  Developing an Effective Therapeutic Relationship. 72

  Using Communication to Engage and Develop Care 74

    Heron's (2001) Six-stage Interventional Analysis. 74

  Recognised Barriers to Effective Communication 75

    Communicating with Children. 76

      Tools to Aid Communication. 76

Notes on Contributors

Claire Agnew van Asch, Senior Nurse – Clinical Practice Development, DipHE in Nursing(Distinction), ENB A24 and 998, Postgraduate Certificate in Continuing Education, MA in Lifelong Education, Doctoral Student

Claire is a Registered Nurse who qualified in 1995 and started her career working within the fields of care of the elderly and acute medical admissions. Claire has always been passionate about supporting staff to be the best that they can be, pioneering a clinical nurse educator role within her Trust in 1998, and since then the rest of her career has been in the field of education, training and practice development, both at the bedside and in the classroom. Claire specialises in preceptorship and is the lead for the practice learning and preceptorship faculties within the School of Nursing and Midwifery Practice. She has been the chair of the East Midlands Preceptorship Group since 2016 and more recently has spent 6 years in the LLR School of Nursing Associates as a module leader for the FDSc Nursing Associate Programme.

Annabel Coulson, Programme Leader LLR FDSc Nursing Associate RN, BA Nursing, PGCert Leadership, PGCert HE with NMC Recordable Teacher, Doctoral Student

Annabel qualified as a Registered Nurse in 1991, having trained within a School of Nursing under an apprenticeship model. Annabel has always had a passion for education and after 16 years in clinical practice, working predominantly in medical wards and intensive care units, moved into an education role. Annabel supported practice learning for nursing students and had a leadership role in curriculum development for pre-registration nursing and mentorship programmes through a close working relationship with the local university. In 2016 Annabel led the development of the Leicester, Leicestershire and Rutland Nursing Associate Programme which remains the only programme designed, delivered and managed within an NHS Trust. As the Programme Leader, Annabel works with a devoted team who ensure that the best interests of the students are at the centre of the programme; the team actively listens to students and this passion is reflected in the pages of this book. Module leaders within the programme have an extensive practice and educational background and are passionate about the programme and the nursing associate and regularly advocate for the role. Annabel's doctoral study focuses on the lived experience of the nursing team in relation to the inclusion of the NA role and it is hoped that this will enable greater exploration of how the role is evolving.

Leigh-Ann Cowell, Module Leader LLR FDSc Nursing Associate RNC, Adv Dip, BMedSci (Hons), PGCertHE

Leigh-Ann is a Module Lead and Lecturer within the LLR School of Nursing Associates, as well as joint lead of induction and pre-programme workshops. She has a passion for teaching and a keen interest in supporting workforce development, ensuring success through the programme. She qualified as a Registered Nurse for Children in 1999 from the University of Sheffield, and worked within paediatric cardiac services in Leicester for the first 15 years of her career. It was here that she found a love for teaching at the bedside and went on to become a clinical educator. Later moving into the Education team within a children's hospice, she played a lead role alongside the matron in introducing the Nursing Associate role into the team, and completing her PGCert in higher education, before moving to her current role.

Jacqueline Elton, Module Leader LLR FDSc Nursing Associate RN, PhD Law, LLM(Distinction), MA, BSc(Hons)

Jacqueline Elton has worked within the UHL for many years in a variety of roles as a clinical nurse, ward sister, matron and deputy head of nursing before moving into education as a module lead on the Nursing Associate Programme. She has a doctorate in law and her special interest is nursing law and ethics which threads through much of her teaching. Jacqueline leads the second-year module Principles of Care Delivery. This module looks at a systems-based approach to anatomy and physiology before going on to look at what happens when care delivery goes wrong.

Marie Knight, Module Leader RN, MSc

Marie is a Registered Adult Nurse with experience in a range of settings, including community nursing, stroke and cardiology, and education roles. Marie is passionate about ensuring patients and carers have equal access to care and support services which are centred around their individual needs which is the focus for her module on the programme. Marie has now retired to spend time with her family.

Colette Orton, Module Leader LLR FDSc Nursing Associate RGN, DPSN, BA(Hons) Cert Ed, PGCHE

Colette has worked in the acute care sector, predominantly in surgical settings, with experience across cardiac intensive care, hepatobiliary, orthopaedic and emergency nursing. Colette developed a passion for teaching and taught in a further education college, then transferred those skills in a post as a clinical nurse educator, working directly with newly registered nurses, healthcare assistants and students from a variety of backgrounds. Colette currently leads on a module that is delivered in the second year of the programme, entitled Team Working and Collaborative Practice. It focuses on the team around the patient and how the nursing associate contributes to the improvement and delivery of high-quality, safe care, as part of the multidisciplinary team in a variety of healthcare settings.

Michelle Richardson, Module Leader LLR FDSc Nursing Associate RNMH MMedSci, DipHE

Michelle is a Registered Mental Health Nurse, qualifying in 2007. Michelle's clinical experience has stretched across Medium and Low secure environments and Psychiatric Intensive Care. Michelle then moved into clinical Education with in Physical acute settings, supporting Adult and Mental Health Student Nurses within clinical practice. Since 2020, she has been a module leader on the programme as well as developing the Mental Health Curriculum across the programme. She has move recently taken on the role of Education Wellbeing Lead, supporting the learning differences and mental health of the students. Outside of the team, Michelle has aligned herself with projects focused on developing the work forces Mental Health knowledge, through her work with the LLR Staff Wellbeing services.

Rose Webster, Module Leader LLR FDSc Nursing Associate RN DHSci, MSc, BSc (Hons)

Rose Webster specialised in cardiac nursing for over 25 years, followed by a decade working in professional development. She has a background in nursing research, focusing on qualitative methods to explore the lived experiences of cardiac patients and their families. Her doctoral thesis studied the experiences of healthcare assistants new to working in an acute hospital trust. Rose leads on the Evidence Based Practice module of the FDSc programme and also has an interest in supporting students to develop academic confidence, particularly with their writing skills.

Acknowledgements

With thanks to Eleanor Meldrum, Deputy Chief Nurse University Hospitals of Leicester, for having confidence in us and for supporting the Leicester, Leicestershire and Rutland Nursing Associate Programme Team to develop a programme that remains one of a kind.

Introduction

The nursing associate role (NA) is still relatively new and is evolving; students studying the Foundation Degree Science (FDSc) Nursing Associate were originally termed 'trainees' to protect the apprenticeship model and to differentiate learners from the student nurse. The Nursing and Midwifery Council (NMC) has now issued guidelines to education providers to clarify the title to be used. The term student nursing associate (SNA) will be used throughout this book.

This book has been written by the Programme Team for the Leicester, Leicestershire and Rutland (LLR) Nursing Associate Programme and is aimed at both students and qualified NAs. The LLR Nursing Associate Programme Team are employed by University Hospitals of Leicester and have been involved in supporting SNAs since the pilot in 2017 (Coulson 2019). This book is the result of experience gained during the development and delivery of the programme and demonstrates the importance of ensuring that the NA role is firmly embedded in practice. The programme team are passionate about the role and supporting the integration of the NA within the nursing workforce. This book provides core content to support students as they embark on their NA journey and insight into the challenges and opportunities of the NA role in today's healthcare system.

The book is divided into nine chapters which explore the development of the role, the importance of professional development and the development of core skills and competencies as outlined by the Nursing and Midwifery Council (NMC 2018). Where appropriate, chapters outline their relationship directly to the Standards of Proficiency and each chapter includes further reading to enable the reader to expand their understanding in relation to their own experiences and practice needs. Chapters are addressed to the reader and a brief outline of each of the chapters and chapter authors is presented here.

Chapter 1: Understanding Your Aprenticeship.
Author: Annabel Coulson

This chapter explores the nature of apprenticeships as a model for learning and the historical context as well as having a more up-to-date look at how apprenticeships can support individuals who may not have had an opportunity to access the more 'traditional' university route. This chapter will support you to understand both your responsibility and your employer's responsibility as an apprentice studying towards your nursing associate registration.

Chapter 2: Embedding the Nursing Associate in Practice.
Author: Jacqui Elton

This chapter will support you to understand the background, training and context for this new role and to explore how this role can and does make a difference. The chapter will examine the background to the role, how it came about and consider some of the controversies and concerns that did and perhaps continue to surround it. We will also look at several examples from across the health and social care platform where this new role has successfully been embedded and is beginning to make that difference.

Chapter 3: Being a Professional: The Importance of 'Scope of Practice'.
Author: Claire Agnew van Asch

This chapter considers the transition to registered practice and the importance of maintaining a professional perspective. It explores the concepts of professionalism and what this means to you. You will reflect on the importance of decision making and evidence-based practice. This chapter introduces several themes that are developed further within the rest of the book.

Chapter 4: Applying Person-centred Approaches to Care.
Author: Leigh-Ann Cowell

This chapter will explore the role of the NA in establishing an early relationship with individuals and sustaining it during the episode of care. Registered NAs will be able to explore different approaches to ensuring a person-centred approach while establishing their role in aspects such as admission and assessment and supporting the development of patient-focused care planning.

Chapter 5: Effective Communication for the Nursing Associate.
Author: Michelle Richardson

This chapter will focus on developing effective communication skills aimed at supporting health individuality, gaining trust and ensuring the patient voice is recognised. The chapter will consider the principles taught during the programme in relation to the NMC Standards (NMC 2018) and how these can be developed. Attention will be paid to the NA role in activities such as breaking bad news, developing a multidisciplinary approach to managing language barriers and developing effective relationships.

Chapter 6: The Nursing Associate and Duty of Care, Candour, Equality and Diversity.
Author: Marie Knight

Duty of care, candour and equality and diversity are concepts that are often discussed when considering nursing and keeping our patients safe but what do they really mean? This is the focus of this chapter, and it will explore these three concepts in more detail, how they interlink, and their relevance to you as a NA.

Chapter 7: The Team Around the Patient.
Author: Colette Orton

This chapter will explore what teamwork and collaborative practice are and how healthcare professionals can deliver safe care and contribute to continuous improvement in services. Nursing associates, by the nature of the role, are ideally placed to deliver and improve care, monitor patient conditions and promote patient safety. They play an important role as members of interdisciplinary teams, collaborating and communicating effectively with nurses, a range of other health and care professionals and lay carers.

Chapter 8: Nursing Associates and the Importance of Being Curious.
Author: Rose Webster

One of the outcomes of the journey to becoming a NA is developing an understanding of the decisions made about care. The theoretical and practical components of your Foundation Degree will have exposed you to some of the latest knowledge and thinking in relation to care delivery. This chapter will encourage you to remain curious and question accepted practice to ensure your patients receive the most effective nursing interventions.

Chapter 9: Supporting Learners: The Role of the Nursing Associate.
Author: Annabel Coulson

As you draw towards the end of your pre-registration programme, you will need to start to consider what it will mean to transition and become a registrant; how this will change your level of responsibility both in terms of your accountability to care for your patients and your responsibility to support others to learn and develop their skills. This chapter will explore this changing role in relation to the support and supervision of learners; you will need to reflect critically on your own experience as a learner to prepare yourself for your future role. This chapter contains useful resources for both the student nursing associate and new registrant.

References

Coulson, A. (2019). Development of an innovative education programme for nursing associates. *Nursing Times* 115 (9): 45–47.

Nursing and Midwifery Council (NMC) (2018). *Standards of Proficiency for Nursing Associates*. London: Nursing and Midwifery Council.

1

Understanding Your Apprenticeship

Annabel Coulson

University Hospitals of Leicester NHS Trust, Leicester, UK

Introduction

You might associate apprenticeships with young people at the start of their careers as an opportunity to gain employment. However, the growing breadth and level of apprenticeships mean that they are popular for anyone considering a career change or further development within a career framework. The Nursing Associate (NA) Apprenticeship (Institute of Apprenticeships Standard ST0827) also enables individuals who have had initial careers as healthcare assistants or healthcare support workers to expand their careers to NMC registration. Some employers will offer opportunities for those who are new to care, or have limited care experience, to enter employment as an apprentice to complete the NA Programme and progress within their nursing careers.

Postregistration opportunities for NAs will also be discussed in this chapter; as a NA there is potential for further development within your role or towards Level 1 registration as a Registered Nurse (RN) by undertaking a further Level 6 Apprenticeship.

This chapter will support you to understand both your responsibility and your employer's responsibility as an apprentice studying towards your NA registration.

Aims of This Chapter

This chapter is relevant to both students and registrants and will be of value to those supporting students in practice.

This chapter aims to:

- provide an overview of the history of nursing education using an apprenticeship model

The Nursing Associate: Stepping into Practice, First Edition. Edited by Annabel Coulson.
© 2025 John Wiley & Sons Ltd. Published 2025 by John Wiley & Sons Ltd.

- explore the benefits and risks of the apprenticeship as an educational concept
- understand the needs of apprentice NAs within the workplace; from this point the apprentice NA will be termed 'student'
- to develop an awareness of some of the challenges that face students and how these may be overcome.

It is recognised that not all students will enter the NA role via the apprenticeship route. This chapter aims to provide those of you completing an apprenticeship with a greater level of understanding of your responsibility and the responsibility of your employer in supporting your development. While this chapter does not link directly to the NMC Standards of Proficiency for NAs, it does discuss the knowledge, skills and behaviours that are assessed as part of the Institute of Apprenticeships Standard (ST0827) and you will see how closely aligned these are to the NMC Standards of Proficiency (NMC 2018a).

The History of Nurse Education and the Apprenticeship Model

Learning how nurse education has evolved will enable you to develop an understanding of some of the challenges and opportunities associated with an apprenticeship model, either during your educational programme or when supporting others. Nurse education has a long history of using an apprenticeship model of delivery and various reports have either promoted the benefits or highlighted the challenges of this model. This section will briefly explore the history of nurse education in the context of apprenticeship delivery to provide a background which will help you to consider how to utilise the apprenticeship model effectively. This is a very brief overview and further reading has been provided at the end of the chapter.

In 1860, Florence Nightingale established the Nightingale Training School for Nurses at St Thomas's Hospital in a bid to create a skilled nursing workforce. The training of nurses, termed 'probationers', aimed to ensure that nurses were knowledgeable and skilled and held the welfare of the patient at the centre of their care. Nurses needed to demonstrate compassion and a genuine interest in the needs of the individual. To develop these skills and attributes, Nightingale believed that training should take place in hospitals and be provided by suitably trained ward sisters and matrons. She advocated for standardised training for all nurses and a syllabus was developed with medical staff and senior nurses to ensure that all probationers at St Thomas's had the required knowledge, skills and behaviours for the delivery of compassionate, person-centred care. You will see many of these early expectations mirrored in the expectations of the apprenticeship standard for NAs and within the NMC Code (NMC 2018b).

Training was delivered using a practical, 'hands-on' approach which maintained the vocational importance of nursing; the role of the ward sister was integral in ensuring that probationers were provided with the knowledge and opportunity to practise under supervision before they could be deemed to be suitably trained. Nurse probationers were provided with their training free of charge and were given a small wage and for this, they were expected to work long hours, study and maintain a level of conduct befitting the nurse role. Developments in nurse education continued based on an apprenticeship model of learning and practical application and this model was seen as best practice by consultants, ward sisters and matrons.

In 1919, the Nurses' Registration Act and the foundation of the General Nursing Council resulted in a legal requirement for the standardisation of nurse training, leading to a national training syllabus and examination. To be entered onto the nursing register, an individual had to successfully complete the standard training and assessment and be deemed of good character.

Nurse education and the need to ensure a supply of suitably trained nurses were discussed and debated over the next 50 years; demand for nurses was influenced by global events such as the lasting effects of the First World War and the increased need for hospital care because of the Second World War. Shortages of nurses has been, and continues to be, debated in terms of ensuring that healthcare has access to the right number of suitably skilled staff able to respond to changes in demand and advances in technology and medical science. The NHS Workforce Plan (2023) identified the need for the correct mix of staff to provide effective and compassionate care while also ensuring highly skilled practitioners who are able to meet the increasing complexity of care needs.

Any discussion relating to the education of nurses must include a balance between ensuring the education needs of those seeking a career in nursing and the needs of those employing a nursing workforce. The apprenticeship model of educating nurses remained popular with senior medical and nursing teams when in the 1960s concerns were identified around the status of students and the priority given to their learning. Advocates for the apprenticeship model recognised the importance of practical skill development and feared that by prioritising academia, this would be lost. At the same time there was a concern that students' learning was being compromised in favour of tasks that could be done by non-registered staff. Students identified that they were working long hours with limited time for study and because of staff shortages, they were not getting the support to practise their new skills. While there were reports suggesting that significant change was needed in nurse education, this change did not start to happen for a long time.

The Briggs Report in 1972 recommended that nurse education be more closely aligned to a university in a bid to protect student status and increase the professional identity of nursing. While it was not until much later that nursing finally moved towards a university-based education, the Briggs Report was responsible for initiating the most significant shift in nurse education since Nightingale (Briggs 1972). Briggs recommended that there should be a single tier of nurse, the RN, as there was a lack of appropriate definition between the RN and Enrolled Nurse (EN) and often this resulted in ENs assuming roles that should be limited to the RN. The development and subsequent demise of the EN are discussed in relation to the new NA role in Chapter 2. You might find further reading of the Briggs Report interesting in relation to the development of the NA role.

In 1992, nurse education moved to a university and was delivered by lecturers and nurse academics; student status was maintained throughout the period of the programme, resulting in the immediate loss of the student workforce.

Considerable debate around how nursing programmes prepare students for the demands of healthcare has existed ever since, with calls to increase the amount of time student nurses spend as part of the workforce. The supernumerary status of nursing students continues to be maintained and it could be viewed that the NA apprenticeship offers the opportunity to have the 'best of both worlds'. The lessons learnt from early apprenticeship models and the transition to university-based education will be discussed in greater detail throughout this chapter.

The NA role was developed to bridge the gap between the HCA and the RN; you may be familiar with this concept but if you are not then you must ensure that you read the Shape of Caring Review (Willis 2015). Willis identified the challenges to nurse education and the intention that a role positioned between HCA and RN will provide improved patient care and create development opportunities for existing HCAs. Apprenticeship offers existing HCAs the ability to learn and gain registration while not restricting earning ability, providing an excellent opportunity for experienced HCAs to gain career progression.

What Is an Apprenticeship?

Apprenticeships have existed for many hundreds of years and can be traced to the craft guilds of the Middle Ages. We have already explored the background of nursing apprenticeships and the changing landscape of nurse education which has resulted in the current programmes being offered across many areas of nursing. An apprenticeship provides you with an opportunity to gain education and training towards a recognised qualification while also earning a wage and being part of a workforce – as an apprentice you are entitled to holiday pay and all the usual benefits associated with employment.

Apprenticeships exist in many different fields and offer a wide range of educational levels, All organisations with an annual pay bill of more than £3 million pay 0.5% of their pay bill into the apprenticeship levy, which is then used as a funding pot to support education and training through apprenticeships. As an apprentice, you will complete a recognised programme of study which is funded using the employer's apprenticeship levy, leaving you with no tuition fees to pay. The NA programme must meet both the NMC Standards of Proficiency (NMC 2018a) and the Institute of Apprenticeship Standards (ST0827).

As an apprentice, you will be expected to actively contribute to the workforce for part of your working week, known as 'on the job' learning, and for at least 20% of the time all apprentices must be able to engage in 'off the job' learning. You will learn many practical skills through working closely with existing registrants, nurses and NAs, and as you progress through your programme you should expect to be able to undertake additional skills with less direct supervision. There are skills, such as medicines administration, which must be directly observed by a registrant until you have your own registration and have completed all your associated competencies. Postregistration development is discussed further later in chapter but the most important consideration for you is how the development and execution of skills learnt during the programme are supported by your own local policy. Ensure that you access these and understand what level of direct or indirect supervision is required, which will ensure that you are maintaining your own professional responsibility and acting within your scope of practice.

The Apprenticeship Standards for Nursing Associates (ST0827)

Apprenticeship Standards are determined by the Institute for Apprenticeships and Technical Education and contain the knowledge, skills and behaviours expected by the role identified by the relevant Standard. These Standards are updated from time to time and the Standard referred to within this chapter is ST0287 NA (NMC 2018a). You should be familiar with this Standard as, ultimately, this is the Standard against which you are assessed.

Your role as a NA is discussed at length throughout this book and this chapter will not repeat this discussion. NA is a protected title and can be used only by someone on part 2 of the NMC register. When you review the Apprenticeship Standard, you will see that the requirements to successfully complete this are initially presented as 'Duties' underpinned by a series of knowledge, skills and behaviours which mirror very closely the Standards set out by the NMC. These will be mapped into your Foundation Degree (FDSc) and to successfully achieve registration, you must complete all components of both the academic award and the Apprenticeship Standards including an integrated end point assessment (EPA).

'On-the-Job' Time

When you embark on your programme, you become a student, and this should be your recognised identity throughout the programme whether you are learning 'on' or 'off' the job. 'On-the-job' learning can seem very challenging as there will be an expectation that you act independently within your scope of practice. Students have experienced this as being treated as a HCA; some of you will relate to this and to being asked whether you are a student or HCA for your shift. You may reflect on some of the challenges identified in the Briggs Report (Briggs 1972) during the 1960s when students reported feeling a heightened expectation that they undertake unskilled work which could be completed by domestic staff while nurses were required to complete increasingly skilled and complex duties. Students felt that their learning was not being protected due to shortages of nursing and domestic staff.

It is both your responsibility and that of your employer through the roles of practice assessor and practice supervisor to ensure that you have suitable support to learn both 'on' and 'off' the job. Newer apprenticeships ensure a level of protected learning through 'off-the-job' learning but it is important that you maintain your development and learning while you are expected to contribute to staffing numbers. Due to the requirements of the NMC for you to complete a certain amount of study and supernumerary time in practice, you will have much less requirement for 'on-the-job' learning than other non-nursing apprenticeships may do; it is important that you know through identification within your off duty when you are required to be part of staffing numbers and when your learning is protected. Each university will manage this differently; typically, when you are away from your primary or 'base' area, you will be 'off the job' and while in your base you may have some protected learning and some 'on the job'. You need to be able to identify this, and it must be recorded to ensure that you complete all requirements for your apprenticeship EPA.

'On-the-job' learning may seem difficult and if you have been a HCA for a long time, you may feel that you are doing many similar roles; this causes frustration and has been reported by several students (King et al. 2020; Dainty et al. 2021). Students in these studies identified the need to be proactive and seek opportunities, so it is important that you are aware of any opportunity that might present itself and you take a questioning approach to care. As a registrant, you will need to provide a rationale and explain the decisions you make around care delivery so while you are a student, ensure that you question and develop a greater understanding of why care is being delivered the way it is. Throughout your programme, you will develop a greater understanding of the human body and what affects how well the body responds to mental and physical illness and disease. Your knowledge will provide a foundation for care and when you are taking part in activities which may have been familiar 'tasks' as a HCA, you now need to think about the implication of each activity for the patient. 'On-the-job' work should not be seen as a time to fall back on activities you are familiar with; instead, you should use this time to think differently and apply your knowledge.

As you become more confident, you should be asking to take greater responsibility for roles which you are able to do with less direct supervision, which may include supervising and educating others and taking responsibility for the complete care of patients with lower dependency needs. Discuss with your practice supervisor and practice assessor how you are going to continue to learn while you are included in the nursing numbers; an action plan or learning agreement may help you with this. Your university will also have specific guidelines about 'on-the-job' learning and may support you to identify specific areas for development.

'Off-the-Job' Learning

This type of learning includes your academic time and theory, and under the requirements of the NMC this constitutes 50% of your overall programme; theory may be made up of study days or seminars, guided learning and self-directed study. Your university will give you the detail around the provision of your academic or theory hours, ensure that you understand the timetable and that you discuss this with your manager; as an apprentice they are supporting your learning both in theory and in practice. As an apprentice, you are also an employee, and you are being paid to attend theory; ensure that you abide by your usual employment responsibility when reporting any sickness and absence from study as this forms part of your contracted hours.

Practice hours constitute the remaining 50% of your programme; protected learning or 'off-the-job' hours must enable you to learn and develop skills while not being included in the nursing establishment of the ward, department or practice area. This means that you should be 'free' to take part in additional activities which you would not normally be able to do because of 'getting the job done'. Students have recognised challenges with 'off-the-job' hours as the conflicting priorities associated with care delivery result in the erosion of dedicated time for learning.

> Student: 'My manager gives me protected learning time, but often this is taken away by senior managers wanting me to complete HCA roles.'

It is impossible to deny that there will be challenges due to the pressures associated with ensuring patients are given the care they need, but it is important that you are supported. Between you, your practice assessor and practice supervisor and your university, you need to determine what activities you need to engage in to support your learning; this will provide structure to your protected learning time and your managers will have a better understanding of how you can relate this to your continuing development. In your area of employment, you may struggle to gain the protected learning time that you are allocated and this can be frustrating, so ensure that you discuss any concern with your manager as soon as you can. You may also have access to a practice learning team who can support you and your manager to protect your learning time and explore opportunities.

> Student: 'In my base area I don't do anything different, I just work as an HCA.'

Seeking support early will avoid this frustration and ensure that you remain focused on the requirements of your programme.

Students have identified that the challenges faced during their pre-registration programme are due to a lack of awareness by managers and peers in relation to their role as a student and their anticipated role on completion (Dainty et al. 2021).

Placements may make up a significant amount of your 'off-the-job' practice hours. On placement, you will gain experiences across all fields of nursing practice, 'in the home', 'close to home' and 'in hospital', and during this time you will need to practise skills which you are familiar with in a different setting. You will also need to explore other aspects of care to allow you a greater understanding of the patient journey, the specialists and teams patients encounter and what support they may have for different needs. As a NA, you will not be limited to a specific field of nursing practice such as adult, child, mental health or learning disability and as such you might want to explore specific aspects of care. For example, a patient needing surgery in adult secondary care who also has a significant learning disability will need additional support; you may want to consider what services are available to support the individual and their family. There will be several specialists and teams involved in any person's care, and your 'off-the-job' hours provide you with the opportunity to explore this. Your practice assessor and practice supervisor are responsible for supporting this development, so discuss this with them and ensure that you are proactive about your learning needs; use of an action plan can help.

As an apprentice, you must ensure that you involve your manager in your experiences; it is important that they are aware of how you are developing and how you are using these experiences to evolve your own practice, so sharing reflections and your practice assessment document will facilitate this. As an employee, you must ensure that you are following your local policy with regard to sickness, absence and annual leave; Failure to do so may result in a disciplinary investigation and failure to meet the NMC Code, leading to a professional conduct concern which will ultimately affect your ability to register with the NMC.

'Off-the-job' hours protect your learning and provide you with the opportunity to practise skills under supervision, but you do remain part of a team and this does not preclude you from being involved in all aspects of care. You need to ensure that you are an active participant and not an observer. It may feel that you are walking a very fine line between being a student and having responsibilities as an employee, which is reflected in the experiences of many students and is something that universities and practice partners are working hard to try and resolve. If you do feel overwhelmed with these competing priorities or feel that your learning is not being effectively supported, you must speak to your manager, your practice assessor and your university and seek out your practice learning team.

Getting the Right Balance

We have discussed the origins of nurse education and the apprenticeship model of education; we have explored some of the opportunities and challenges associated with the NA apprenticeship. As a relatively new role, the NA is evolving, and understanding of the training programme is growing amongst current RNs and student nurses. Students embarking on the NA programme find that the challenges of balancing being a worker and a student overwhelming. The challenges of having a family and commitments outside the programme add to this pressure (Coghill 2018).

As you embark on, continue with or try and support others on their programme, it is important that you understand these challenges and how to manage them. As an apprentice, you need to ensure that you are meeting the academic and practice demands of the programme while also maintaining a healthy work–life balance. Students who decide not to continue often do so because of challenges associated with trying to find the right balance. Some preparation prior to starting the programme may help you to minimise the risk of leaving because of this conflicting demand. If you are considering how to best support a student, it is important to recognise that they often have family commitments and other priorities, so getting to know your student and supporting them to seek appropriate help may reduce the risk of them leaving the programme.

As a student, make sure that you are prepared before you start. Ask yourself the following questions.

- What do you know about the programme you are studying?
  - Do you understand the commitments to study outside your normal working week? This could include reading, preparing academic assignments and ensuring that you are reflecting on your practice.
  - Do you understand the academic level you will need to study and write at, and what challenges might this give you?

- Are there any anticipated significant life events in the next two years? You will not be able to predict everything but make sure that you are as aware as possible of anything that may impact on your ability to commit to the programme at the level expected of you.
- Have you planned for the programme?
  - Make a weekly planner of everything you do during the week: work pattern, family commitments, leisure activities, managing your home – shopping, cooking, etc. Now look at the additional expectations of the programme and how you will fit these in. If you have to give anything up to be able to manage the programme, will you be happy to do this?

Postregistration Opportunities

So far, this chapter has looked at the challenges and opportunities that come with being an apprentice and how you can manage your pre-registration journey. We will now look at the potential opportunities post registration; you may want to return to this later in your programme.

As a NA, you are registered on the NMC register. As you are aware, the NA is a generic role which means that your programme has provided you with the underpinning knowledge to work in all fields of nursing practice. During your programme, you will have been based in an area which may have focused you towards one field of practice; you now have the flexibility to move into different areas. Now that you have registered, you will need to consider how you want to develop within your career.

Preceptorship

All new registrants must complete a period of preceptorship. The new Preceptorship Standards for nurses and NAs were published in 2022 to ensure that all new registrants continue to be supported to embed their role and increase confidence in their role (NHS England 2022). Preceptorship should last for one year and include dedicated time to learn and be supported. As a new registrant, you will have a preceptor who will support you in your new role. Preceptorship will include a structured programme to facilitate your integration into the nursing workforce. You will need to spend dedicated time with your preceptor who will discuss your career progression so to prepare for preceptorship, make sure you think about your career development.

What Are Postregistration Opportunities?

At the point of registration, you will have completed all the skills and competencies identified in the NMC Standards. While this is your initial scope of practice, you now can develop a range of skills to complement your role. Your local policy will dictate the boundaries to your practice, and it is your responsibility to make yourself familiar with your own organisation's policies. Preceptorship will support you to consolidate the skills developed during your programme and during this time, you should start to plan your development beyond registration. Development of skills will be supported through local education and training and competence will be assessed using your organisation's educational framework. You should not feel pressured or rushed to expand your skills; ensure that you feel confident to expand beyond your initial registration and talk to your preceptor about how you want to develop within your role.

There are differences between universities and organisations as to the opportunities available post registration; the information below reflects some of the possible development pathways, so explore within your area to see what is available and discuss this during preceptorship and with your manager at your appraisal.

The NA programme offers a recognised route to RN development; many universities offer programmes so explore what is offered locally. When you consider developing as an RN, you will need to determine what field of practice to focus on. This will mainly be dependent on your area of practice but may also be influenced by other factors such as personal interest; for example, you might work in an adult area but want to develop your mental health skills and support patients with mental health concerns.

Registration as a NA offers you several opportunities for development within your career; the most frequently discussed is the route towards RN. Many Trusts and organisations supporting the NA role also support ongoing progression to RN through an apprenticeship route, often referred to as the 'top-up'. However, you should recognise that by going down the RN route, you are changing your role. Rather than thinking of the RN route as being a 'top up', you should think of this as a transition to a different role.

When you undertake the RN, you will move from a generic role, encompassing all fields of nursing practice, to one which is more focused within your area of interest or practice. It will be up to you and your manager to determine the most appropriate registration from adult, child, mental health and learning disability. Typically, these programmes are between 18 months and two years in length, and you will need to be supported by your employer, explore what is available locally and discuss this during your appraisal. While you undertake the RN development programme, you need to ensure that you maintain your NA registration and complete any revalidation which may be required by the NMC.

The NHS Long Term Workforce Plan recognises the importance of embedding the NA role within practice and identifies the need for a rapid and sustained increase in the number of NAs within the workforce. To retain NAs within practice, development opportunities are needed within the role itself, so some universities have developed a bespoke suite of modules enabling NAs to complete a BSc and expand their knowledge and skills within their role. Typically, NA roles sit at Band 4 under Agenda for Change but when the role was initially developed, there was no given 'ceiling' to the role and expansion of knowledge and skills can result in posts at higher banding. Concerns about role substitution have been prevalent within some social media posts and discussion papers but there is no evidence that this has happened, and the role was not established to replace nurses but rather to enrich knowledge and skills throughout the nursing team.

Whether you choose to develop your career through RN transition or through a BSc, you need to consider your options as you progress through your initial preceptorship and develop a personal development plan. Some organisations will have internal development programmes which are part of the Continuing Professional Development (CPD) for all RNs, NAs and midwives. These programmes include the development of specific skills and knowledge around subjects such as dementia or support for end of life. All organisations will have a preceptorship programme which will help you to consolidate the skills developed through your pre-registration programme, so ensure that you discuss your plans and ideas for development with your preceptor and manager.

Chapter Summary

This chapter has explored the origin of nurse apprenticeships and considered the context of nurse education over the past 100 years. You have had the opportunity to reflect on this in relation to your developing role as a NA. An apprenticeship may have offered you a very personal opportunity to develop into a nursing role you may have thought impossible. If you have started your NA programme, you have commenced your journey towards a rewarding career as a registrant; as a previous healthcare support worker, you will be extending your skills.

The chapter has explored the challenges associated with being an employee while at the same time learning and developing more specialist skills. The rest of this book will discuss the core components of the NMC Standards on which all NA programmes are based.

References

Briggs, A. (1972). *Report of the Committee on Nursing*. London: HMSO.

Coghill, E. (2018). An evaluation of how trainee nursing associates (TNAs) balance being a 'worker' and a 'learner' in clinical practice: an early experience study. Part 1/2. *British Journal of Healthcare Assistants* 12 (6): 280–286.

Dainty, A.D., Barnes, D., Bellamy, E. et al. (2021). Opportunity, support and understanding: the experience of four early trainee nursing associates. *British Journal of Healthcare Assistants* 15 (6): 284–291.

King, R., Ryan, T., Wood, E. et al. (2020). Motivations, experiences and aspirations of trainee nursing associates in England: a qualitative study. *BMC Health Services Research* 20 (1): 802.

NHS England (2022). National Preceptorship Framework for Nursing. www.england. nhs.uk/wp-content/uploads/2022/10/B1918_i_National-preceptorship- framework-for-nursing-10-October-2022.pdf

NHS England (2023). *NHS Long Term Workforce Plan*. London: NHS England.

Nursing and Midwifery Council (NMC) (2018a). *Standards of Proficiency for Nursing Associates*. London: Nursing and Midwifery Council.

Nursing and Midwifery Council (NMC) (2018b). *The Code. Professional Standards of Practice and Behaviour for Nurses, Midwives and Nursing Associates*. London: Nursing and Midwifery Council.

Willis, P. (2015). *Raising the Bar. Shape of Caring: A Review of the Future Education and Training of Registered Nurses and Care Assistants*. London: Health Education England.

2

Embedding the Nursing Associate in Practice

Jacqueline Elton

University Hospitals of Leicester NHS Trust, Leicester, UK

Introduction

If you are reading this it is possible that you are a nursing associate (NA), are thinking about becoming one or maybe just want to have a better understanding of what the background, training and context are for this new role. You may also want to see how this role can and does make a difference to how the nursing team are able to provide holistic, person-centred care.

In this chapter we will examine the background to the role, how it came about and consider some of the controversies and concerns that did and perhaps continue to surround it. We will also look at several examples from across the health and social care platform where this new role has successfully been embedded and is beginning to make that difference.

Aims of This Chapter

- To gain an understanding of how the role came about and some of the controversies surrounding it.
- To gain an understanding of the difficulties surrounding the introduction of a new role.
- To gain an appreciation of how the role can be integrated into care using real case studies.

Related NMC Standards

- *Platform 1 Being an Accountable Professional:* NAs act in the best interests of people, putting them first and providing nursing care that is person centred, safe and compassionate. They always act professionally and use their knowledge and experience to make evidence-based decisions and

The Nursing Associate: Stepping into Practice, First Edition. Edited by Annabel Coulson.
© 2025 John Wiley & Sons Ltd. Published 2025 by John Wiley & Sons Ltd.

solve problems. They recognise and work within the limits of their competence and are responsible for their actions.

- *Platform 6 Contributing to Integrated Care:* NAs contribute to the provision of care for people, including those with complex needs. They understand the roles of a range of professionals and carers from other organisations and settings who may be participating in the care of a person and their family, and their responsibilities in relation to communication and collaboration.

In January 2019 the first qualified NA registrants joined the health and social care workforce (NMC 2019). These were the first of the new registered nursing role and they were and are regulated by the Nursing and Midwifery Council (NMC) which is the regulatory body for nurses, NAs, midwives and health visitors in the UK. The NA was introduced in response to several pressures, the most important being the actual and predicted shortage of nurses and qualified care staff in the UK. The recommendation that a new role be added to the nursing workforce to bridge the gap between the registered nurse (RN) and the healthcare assistant (HCA) was set out in the Willis Review (Willis 2015) and would seem on the face of it a simple answer: a gap has been identified and there are individuals out there who are keen to advance their careers and fill that gap. However, as we will see, the introduction of a new role is often problematic, with several possible obstacles making the introduction and embedding of the role far from simple.

This chapter has two distinct sections – the first part considers the context of the change and possible resistance to the role, including concerns over reinventing the state enrolled nurse (SEN) and that the NA role is in effect 'nursing on the cheap' (Harrold 2016). The second part of the chapter will look at successful introduction of the role using case studies to demonstrate how the role can successfully embed within practice, thus improving patient care and increasing opportunity for individuals who want to undertake nurse training but are reluctant/unable (for whatever reason) to go via the traditional university route.

Why the Need for a New Role?

A newspaper headline in 2016 asked the question, *The NHS is desperately short of nurses. Could a new role hold the answer?* (Thomas 2016), before going on to explain the intention to create the NA role. The level of that shortage is clear if one considers the most recent vacancy figures at the time of writing. These indicated there were 34,709 posts vacant within the RN staff group, equating to a vacancy rate of 8.7% as at 31 December 2023 (NHS Digital 2024). To give this context, it means that approximately 1 in every 11 posts is unfilled.

While there is consensus that there is a shortage of trained nurses, it is important not to simply take these figures at face value. For example, what do qualified nurse shortages mean for patients? Ball and Griffiths (2022) undertook a meta-analysis of 35 studies which met their inclusion criteria and amongst their conclusions there was:

- strong evidence from several large observational studies that lower nurse staffing levels were associated with higher rates of death and falls

- strong evidence that higher nurse staffing is associated with reduced length of stay and lower readmission rates
- similar but less consistent evidence on infections.

It is suggested that a shortage of qualified nurses leads to poorer patient outcomes. It also should be noted that the vacancies are not evenly distributed, with more vacancies in some areas such as mental health and learning disability (Jones-Berry 2019), but also the data from which this information is collected are arguably not robust. Jones-Berry (2019) notes that 'without consistent, unambiguous staffing data, it's difficult to gauge exact nurse numbers and vacancies'.

Although a shortage of trained nurses is one of the key drivers behind the NA role, there are other reasons behind its introduction. The origin of the role can be seen as arising from several high-profile reports into care failures within the NHS (Francis 2013; Berwick 2013) which identified the need for high-quality compassionate care. In response to these, Lord Willis was asked to lead a review into the appropriateness and effectiveness of nurse education within both health and social care: the Raising the Bar – Shape of Caring review (Willis 2015). Several threads were identified in this paper and a key one for this chapter was that:

> *HEE should explore with others the need to develop a defined care role... that would act as a bridge between the unregulated care assistant workforce and the registered nursing workforce (p.39)*

and further that alternative routes into nursing should be available for care assistants who wished to undertake training.

Another important component of this was that funding should be reviewed to ensure that those who wished to access NA training could do so without being prevented by fear of university fees or of having to lose income by giving up their jobs to become full-time students. This question was ultimately addressed by making one of the routes into NA training an apprenticeship, therefore widening access as Lord Willis recommended.

While it is undeniable that there is a shortage of nurses and that the NA role is seen as being part of the answer, the introduction of the role is far from a knee-jerk reaction to those shortages.

The chapter introduction noted the idea that this route may be appealing for those who do not wish to study via the traditional university route, which is worth considering in more detail. The traditional route into nurse training is a three-year university degree, typically requiring at least two (usually three) A-levels or equivalent qualifications at level 3, plus supporting GCSEs (NHS Careers n.d.) to gain entry. The three-year programme means being a full-time student, and although there is some financial support available, tuition fees and living expenses accumulate. The NA role is a two-year Foundation degree, and the entry requirements are GCSEs grade 9–4 (A–C) in maths and English, or Functional Skills Level 2 in maths and English (NHS Careers n.d.). The NA qualification is a standalone registration which can also be used as a stepping stone to become an RN. As this is typically via the apprenticeship route, the student NA can continue to work and take a salary, while not accumulating tuition fees.

With the opening of this alternative route for HCAs to enter education, it seems reasonable to speculate that such individuals will often have roots within an area, so may have children at the local school and have established support and friendship networks in the area. As such, HCAs wishing to register as NAs with established roots seem more likely to stay in the area, even if they move wards/locations after qualification – thus improving retention. This is important as poor retention of recruited staff is an important issue within the workforce. Given how new the role is, it is not yet possible to evidence this point, but logically to the author it makes sense.

For individuals following this career path, the new role will allow career development for those wishing to specialise as an NA and allow those who wish to go on and undertake RN training a career path for HCAs that did not exist even five years ago.

Is the NA a Reinvention of the SEN?

Some of you reading this will be unaware of the SEN role, but it is arguably important to understand what happened with that role as there are parallels with the NA role. The SEN role was introduced by the Nurses Act (1943), in response to staff shortages and the perceived need to improve the numbers of trained nurses during World War 2. The SEN followed a two-year course of training and on qualifying was placed on the 'Roll' which was maintained and administered by the General Nursing Council (GNC), a predecessor of the NMC, in contrast to the state registered nurse[1] (SRN) who undertook a three-year programme of training and was placed on the 'Register'.

Is the NA reinventing the SEN? The background and context surrounding both the SEN and NA role will be considered to demonstrate that this concern is misplaced in that the NA role takes many of the strengths of the SEN role, but adds a range of distinctions that will give the role a very clear identity of its own. It will also be noted that the NA reintroduces a second level of nurse registration which has been and continues to be used successfully in many other countries.

As the first cohort of NAs were coming close to completing their education in 2018, this sentiment regarding the reinvention of the SEN and 'nursing on the cheap' was outlined in an article in the *Guardian* newspaper (Brindle 2018) where several questions were asked about the NA role, one of which was whether the role was simply a reinvention. This needs closer examination as although it could be argued that there are similarities, there are also fundamental differences and, importantly, the SEN role was not removed because it was seen as having been unsuccessful. Indeed, the role was introduced in 1943 and the SEN was the backbone of many care environments for the next 40 years until numbers began to decrease after the cessation of SEN training in the 1990s. In 1992–1993 almost a quarter of

---

[1] The SRN qualification was replaced by the registered general nurse (RGN) in the 1980s, which subsequently became the registered nurse or RN.

qualified nurses were SENs, with that figure dropping to a fifth of all qualified nurses by 1997 (Seccombe et al. 1997, p. ix).

Before moving on to the SEN role specifically, it is worth considering a recent review and thematic analysis undertaken by Lucas et al. (2021). This review focused on the perspectives of healthcare professionals on second-level nursing roles in several countries. Although the SEN role was sometimes controversial in the UK, it is important to note that many other countries also have a second-level nursing role, which in many cases is well established. Examples include the licenced practical nurse and registered practical nurse in the USA and Canada, and the enrolled nurse in both Australia and New Zealand. The roles in these countries tend to focus on care of the more stable and less acutely unwell patients under the supervision of the RN (Lucas et al. 2021).

The review undertaken by Lucas et al. (2021) identified several key themes regarding the role of the second-level nurse, both positive and negative, but for the purpose of this chapter, those of relevance are as follows.

- There was ambiguity between first- and second-level roles; the authors noted it could be difficult to spot the difference and that other healthcare professionals were unclear as to the extent of the second-level roles.
- The role was efficient but the perception was that such roles were limited in their scope with limited opportunity for career progression and limited autonomy within the role.

These issues have been impacting the second-level registered role for the past several decades, particularly in relation to the lack of role clarity.

The UKCC (predecessor organisation to the NMC) stated that it 'impose(d) no arbitrary boundaries between the role of the first and second level registered practitioner' (UKCC 1988 cited in Seccombe et al. 1997). But the reality was very different, with access to more senior posts being largely blocked for SENs (McGough and McGough 1998). This disparity seems to have arisen at least in part due to the interpretation of Rule 18(2) of the Nurses, Midwives and Health Visitors Rule Approval Order 1983 statutory instrument No 873 which sets out the role and responsibilities of the EN. The key sections within the Rule stated the EN should:

- a. Assist in carrying out comprehensive observation of the patient and help in assessing her care requirements.
- b. Develop skills to enable her to assist in the implementation of nursing care under the direction of a person registered in Part 1, 3, 5 or 8 of the register [registered nurse].
- c. Accept delegated nursing tasks.
   (SI1983/873)

Although the language used is of its time, with the nurse being referred to as 'her' all the way through, the point is that 18(2) was clear that the EN worked under the supervision of the RN. However, the more contentious element of this was that 18(2) was at the point of registration and did not make any provision for the EN doing additional training or gaining extra skills, which is presumably the point the UKCC was making about promotion not being blocked.

Lauder and Roxburgh (2006) consider how the demise of the SEN occurred in parallel with the implementation of Project 2000 and the move to the new more academic nurse education which put all RNs on a more equal footing with other university-educated allied health professionals (AHPs). It is argued that this context is important in that a very clear difference between the EN and the NA emerges at this point. EN training was a two-year practically based programme with the written examination being via a multi-choice paper. The education programme for the new NA role still has the strong practical element, but registered NAs will have a Foundation degree and as such a programme of education which, as with the RN programme, aims to inculcate critical reasoning.

Potential Difficulties with the Introduction of New Roles

Halse et al. (2018) undertook a literature review on the introduction of new roles in healthcare, identifying seven key factors which should be considered when introducing new roles.

- Robust workforce planning
- Well-defined scope of practice
- Wide consultation and engagement with stakeholders
- Strong leadership
- An education programme that mirrors patient need
- Adequate resources for work-based learning
- Supervision by a skilled clinical educator
  (Halse et al. 2018, p. 35)

The NA role is not the only new or extended role to be introduced into healthcare over the past decades and it would seem logical to presume that issues which have impacted the previous changes are likely to be replicated with this role. Gray et al. (2010) undertook research regarding the introduction of the physician's assistant (PA) role into anaesthetic departments in the UK, and their finding was that barriers to the acceptance of the role included:

- lack of clarity and confusion about the role
- concerns that it encroached on existing roles.

These findings do not just apply to the PA role. Schindel et al. (2017), considering the expansion of the role of the pharmacist, noted the same issues and more recently Lam et al. (2018) made the same observations in relation to the introduction of a new anaesthesia assistant role in Canada.

While none of these papers was looking at the introduction of the NA role into UK hospitals, there is no reason to believe the same concerns would not arise. This is supported by the findings of King et al. (2020) and Coghill (2018) where both small-scale studies identified the need for role clarity as this was seen as a barrier. King et al. (2020) noting that 'TNAs experienced widespread role ambiguity, both personally and within their organisations'.

Understanding of the Role

A point which should not be underestimated, which is hopefully self-limiting, is that there are still relatively few NAs in comparison to the number of RNs. This, at least in the short term, makes the understanding of the role more limited simply because many RNs will not have worked with NAs. There are some 622,897 RNs and midwives able to practise in the UK, but only about 10,500 NAs (NMC 2023), so NAs currently represent a tiny percentage of the qualified register.

A thought-provoking aside came up in comments at a NA conference held at this author's hospital. Several qualified NAs suggested that rather than having the title NA to distinguish them from the SEN, they should be titled EN as it was their perception that the EN title and role has a degree of both public and professional understanding and comprehension that the new role does not currently enjoy.

The Reality of the NA Role

Noting the points made in the first section of this chapter relating to the theoretical barriers and potential hazards in introducing a new role, what is the real experience of both managers looking to introduce and embed the role and of NAs living the role?

The vignettes which follow do not represent a scientific evaluation of the role but rather show how the role introduction can and has been handled to ensure that the role can be an effective part of the workforce and, for the individuals, shows the range of possibilities for the role and for those individuals. The vignettes do not represent staff from all specialisms or settings; they come from a range of settings where the role has been adopted in a way that is viewed locally as being successful.

Annabel – Programme Lead

While the focus of the vignettes is how the role has embedded in the 'real world', to give this context it is perhaps useful to first gain a perspective on how the original authors of a nursing associate Foundation degree in science (FDSc) saw this happening. Also, we look at how the course design and organisation was intended to ensure that this role had a clear identity and was able to embed, so in effect providing a link between the theory of introducing a new role and the reality of trying to ensure the implementation was a success.

When I was asked to set up the pilot NA programme in 2016, the notion that this would bridge the gap between the HCA and the RN was clear – but the reality of how to create this new role such that there was understanding and support for the role was less clear. We were setting up a unique model for the programme with a university-approved degree based within the practice setting working across the whole health economy within the county. There have now been 11 cohorts who have graduated, a further six cohorts are on the programme with an intended intake of 150 trainees over three cohorts a year from 2023 onwards. Eleven cohorts of NAs have graduated from the School, and the role is becoming increasingly well embedded in practice.

At the time we were looking at a pilot project with the local university to set up a programme around the HEE curriculum framework. We got the template for this in November 2016 and basically the programme was written at speed around this template, with our first cohort starting in early 2017. It was unbelievable how quickly we moved from intention to people actually starting. My vision was that this new role would open the way to new ways of working.

Deadlines were tight as at the point we started, we did not know the role was going to be registered with the NMC, and it was not until 2018 that we, along with the rest of the country, knew that the role was going to be registered. While we were delighted that the role was going to get the recognition and governance we felt it deserved, it did mean a flurry of activity to ensure that the course and trainees were compliant with the requirements for registration – we had to demonstrate that our students' competencies mapped directly across on the NMC competencies – they did!

Given the speed with which we started this, it did make the early days quite problematic in terms of getting the ward managers on board to support the programme and to put forward HCAs for it. This was made possible in part because of the vision of the then Chief Nurse and her vision for a more flexible workforce. While it has not always been straightforward, I would say that these early hurdles have been overcome successfully.

While I am not sure that the vision for a new way of working has been completely fulfilled, I do think that fundamental changes and broadening of the nursing workforce give great development opportunities to HCAs who would otherwise have no avenue for advancement.

As I was working on setting up this role, one of the things which surprised me was the gap between the role of the HCA and the RN, and my perception is that this gap is continuing to widen as the RN role becomes more technical. One of the concerns with the new NA role was that it could go the way of the old SEN qualification and the lack of role clarity would ultimately result in the demise of the role as it became swallowed up by the HCA at one end and the RN at the other.

However, I think by developing the role of the NA as being the knowledgeable bedside doer, who bridges the gap between the task-focused HCA and the more technical RN role, we can and have developed a very clear role identity which gives the basis for future development. We are already seeing NAs doing their RN training but as a knowledgeable doer, the great opportunity for the role is to develop as the bedside specialist.

With the new workforce staffing plan the sky is the limit for the role – but we do need to make sure as nurses that we lead and guide that development.

Jenny – Senior Nurse Manager Acute Hospital Inpatient Setting

The need for strong leadership when introducing new roles was identified in the Halse paper discussed previously. This vignette precisely considers that, looking at how strong leadership has enabled the role to become embedded in acute inpatient areas within a large teaching hospital.

When we first became aware of the role being introduced and were approached about nominating experienced HCAs for the course, we were initially wary, but that was about trying to understand the role. As we had greater clarity around what the role could do, we looked at it as an opportunity. We had high levels of vacancies within our service, and despite efforts at recruitment were not able to rectify this. As the senior team, we looked on this as an opportunity but there was a clear need to ensure that the ward sisters were engaged as the reality would be that they and their teams were going to be the ones to make this work. The idea/plan to recruit NAs from existing experienced HCAs was discussed at the Professional Nurse forums within the services to engage these ward sisters.

We saw this as a huge opportunity for some of our most able HCAs who had potential but either did not have the academic qualifications to access the RN degree and/or were unable to afford to give up work to go to university.

An internal advert then went out to recruit the first tranche of trainee NAs. There was a lot of interest and the first three who went forward all completed the course successfully and are now undertaking the transition course to RN. The service now has a steady stream of HCAs accessing the training, most of whom stay within the service.

In the first tranche, one of the HCAs had to move ward as we were unable to support her adequately on the base ward. With hindsight we realised this was actually a really positive move as it means the trainee has a fresh start as their colleagues do not view them as an HCA. Within the service, we do not advocate that HCAs do move wards once they start their course.

While role clarity is still sometimes an issue, this is now less common but there is still the need for ongoing reinforcement/clarification. There was uncertainty at the time, so the senior nursing management team ensured they were available personally to support both the trainees and the staff working with and supporting them.

One of the points around the role which really served to get the ward sisters on board was the realisation that as an NA cannot be left as the second trained nurse on a shift, it means there will always be a minimum of three registered staff on duty – which means better care for our patients. As things are, currently roughly 10% of the registered staff on the wards with NAs are NAs.

The leadership provided in this area saw a very clear problem relating to difficulty recruiting and retaining RNs and that the NA role was part of a possible solution to enable this to happen by giving clear and explicit support to the role and to the staff who would be working with the NAs to ensure understanding in a way that enabled the role to embed. They also very clearly saw the advantages for HCAs who had the desire and ability to advance their careers.

Claire and Amanda – Community NAs

The issues previously noted around lack of understanding of the role come across clearly in this vignette, but even clearer is the notion that the life experience and education of the NA mean that they can exercise control over how that role embeds, thus making for potentially safer, more effective practitioners.

Claire and Amanda work as recently qualified NAs in a community setting providing care for adult patients. Their list of 'tasks' is extensive and makes it easy to see the differences between the HCA and the NA and the differences in scope of practice of the NA and RN roles. Within their roles, Amanda and Claire:

- administer and monitor patients receiving complex insulin regimes
- undertake complex wound care
- administer medications via a range of routes including IM/SC and patches
- undertake routine catheter changes for both men and women and change suprapubic catheters
- contribute to the assessment of patients.

They have a high degree of autonomy undertaking these tasks, but do not have an identified case load of their own. This, coupled with the fact that they contribute to rather than lead on assessment of patients, highlights a key difference between the NA and RN.

Much of nursing care now is driven by protocols and policies. The function of a policy is to ensure consistent and safe care regarding whatever that policy applies to. Policies will always state what staff groups they apply to or cover. With the NA role being a new one, Amanda and Claire realised that many of the policies in their area did not currently include the NA role. They became aware of a mismatch between two existing policies towards the end of the course, where one policy stated that insulin administration was not within scope of practice for NAs and a second policy said that staff with pre-existing skills should maintain these. They highlighted this discrepancy to a senior manager who asked them how they could address this.

Claire and Amanda subsequently wrote a proposal for the review of all policies which potentially may relate to the NA role. This has been shared with and presented to senior nurse managers within the area and been well received. Having raised their profile by highlighting this concern and being tasked with addressing the issue, other opportunities have also arisen for Claire and Amanda, including presenting at recruitment events and being asked to review and be included in the formulation of NA-specific preceptorship guidelines.

Claire and Amanda have not only embedded their role but are facilitating the embedding of the role for the NAs who follow them in this setting, and by doing this the impact of role is clear.

Louise – Trainee Nurse Associate Acute Inpatient Trust

Louise is an experienced HCA who is now approaching the end of the FDSc and will be registering as an NA in the next couple of months. Her base throughout her training has been an acute inpatient area within a teaching Trust. This vignette illustrates both how challenging the embedding of the role can be, but also how the role can also embed within the person during their development. Louise is approaching qualification and was asked to reflect on how undertaking her NA training had changed her and how she now looks at patient care and the learner experience.

I think that the biggest change for me is in my ability to look at things critically and to challenge. I now look at things and ask myself 'Is this the right thing for the patient? Is the planned action the best option for that patient and is it according to the policy or guideline?'. I had always wanted to learn but what I now have is a sense of professional curiosity – I keep asking myself 'What can we improve?'.

Throughout my training I have had some really good placements and some which are not so good; for both of these I have tried to take away both the positives and the negatives. If the placement was not as good as it could have been, then what can I do to ensure that a learner who works with me does not have that same poor experience? I do this by ensuring I build a relationship with that learner to both support them and enable them to access good learning experiences. Something I would like to look at once I qualify is the idea of the TNA link role – so a qualified NA leading and co-ordinating the support of future TNAs in a given area, I have discussed this with my ward sister and she is supportive of the idea.

I do think there is still some confusion about the role at ward level, but that is something that I can help to change.

Louise pinpoints a particular point midway through the course when she felt something changed in how she saw herself and the role.

I had just started a new placement in an unfamiliar area where patients were sicker than I was used to. I was very anxious as to whether or not I could look after these patients, but then I realised that I could when I applied everything I had learned in the preceding year – and realising I could apply what I had learnt and manage in unfamiliar situations gave me a confidence boost and it was like a switch had flicked on.

From that point forward I realised I was a safe nurse in practice with the ability to apply what I know for the benefit of both patients and colleagues.

The first time I really challenged something I saw was when I was working in a paediatric area where I could not understand why blood pressures were not being routinely taken. I asked the staff who said 'We don't do them'. I asked the ward sister who said 'Yes we do', then I checked the policy which says you can depending on your clinical judgement. After I raised this query with the ward team, the sister confirmed the position with the rest of the team. I knew I had made a difference then.

For me the whole two years have been the most eye-opening journey, one I never thought I would get to make because I could not afford to give up work to go to university. By entering nursing through this apprenticeship route, I am now working towards my dream job.

For Louise a key ability gained through her training was a recognition of her own skills and of both the need and the ability to ask 'Why?'. Why is something done in a particular way? Is that the right way? Skills that are essential for any registered healthcare practitioner.

Steph and Sonal – Nursing Associates Supporting and Developing Other Nurse Associates

While for some NAs, the move to RN is logical and possibly part of the career plan, for many NAs there is a desire to develop and grow within the role. This vignette addresses exactly that issue, looking at the experiences and plans of Sonal and Steph, two NAs who are both looking to develop their careers into education, supporting the development of both them and their peers.

Both Steph and Sonal qualified as NAs in the last couple of years and having consolidated their experience in their base areas, have moved into education in the last few months.

SONAL   I could see the need to support the trainees, my background was acute assessment, and having completed my NA course I could see how the variable levels of supervision and support made a huge difference. Some supervisors were brilliant and others were not. My experience of differing levels of supervision in the course of my training made the move into my current post logical – I want to ensure trainees are given the support we were not always able to access.

Some of my more unexpected learning is around how much you can also learn from other members of the teams, of any grade. You learn to advocate for your trainees; as an HCA or whilst I was doing my NA course, I thought of ward sisters or matrons as intimidating, but having met with them when I am supporting learners, they are eager to find out how to better

> support learners and to better understand the role. I would say now managers look to us to help support their learner.
>
> STEPH   My background was quite specialist working in renal, so now I am constantly learning by being exposed to all the different areas our trainees work in. The reason I chose to train as an NA is that I know that this role can make a difference, and by not getting pulled away into management or into 'organisational politics' which can be the case for many RNs, I can continue to develop and learn within my role.
>
> For the development of the NA role more broadly, I think that we need to reach a point where there is a critical mass of NAs on the wards – at the moment you still meet members of staff who are unclear as to the role because they do not work with NAs regularly – we need to reach a point where the majority of staff in all areas can say 'Yes I work with NAs regularly'. At that point, understanding of the role and its development will be clearer.

Both Steph and Sonal are currently undertaking Level 6 modules as part of a BSc (Hons) in Professional Clinical Practice at the local university as part of their continuing professional development and are clear on the advantages this brings.

We are studying with all levels of registered practitioners including ward sisters, matrons and other senior nurses, which means we can fly the flag for the role. You get a sense of empowerment accessing this sort of programme, the feeling of 'I am good enough to be here'. As access to specialist programmes grows, NAs will have the ability to develop into areas that interest them, for example tissue viability, diabetes, etc. In short, we can be a role model for other NAs showing that you can develop and grow within your role.

This vignette shows the ability of an individual to develop into the role in such a way as to make a difference to both peers and ultimately to patients.

Chapter Summary

Is the NA role simply nursing on the cheap and a reinvention of the SEN? While elements of this will be addressed further in this book, those writing this book would suggest not. The SEN role or its equivalent continues to be used successfully in many countries, and a key difference between the SEN and NA role in England is the level of training and qualification to be able to practise as an NA.

Nursing has moved to being an all-degree profession over the last 20 years and the introduction of the NA role continues in that same vein with the requirement to hold an FDSc. But nursing is not just about qualifications – it is about the delivery of care and the desire to deliver that care at the bedside. As the vignettes demonstrated, NAs both in the community and in acute hospitals are seen by managers as an essential part of the workforce and equally as importantly are seen by themselves as part of the wider nursing family who can make a real difference.

References

Ball, J.E. and Griffiths, P. (2022). Consensus Development Project (CDP): an overview of staffing for safe and effective nursing care. *Nursing Open* 9 (2): 872–879.

Berwick Report (2013). *A Promise to Learn – A Commitment to Act*. London: National Advisory Group on Safety of Patients.

Brindle, D. (2018). Nursing associates: will they become a cheap substitute for nurses? www.theguardian.com/healthcare-network/2018/mar/06/nursing-associates-cheap-substitute-nurses

Coghill, E. (2018). An evaluation of how trainee nursing associates (TNAs) balance being a 'worker' and a 'learner' in clinical practice: an early experience study. *British Journal of Healthcare Assistants* 12 (6): 280–286.

Francis, R. (2013). *Report of the Mid Staffordshire NHS Foundation Trust Public Inquiry HC 497*. London: Stationery Office.

Gray, M., Smith, F., McKeown, D. et al. (2010). Integrating physician assistants into the practice setting. *Nursing Management* 17 (7): 23–27.

Halse, J., Reynolds, L., and Attenborough, J. (2018). Creating new roles in healthcare: lessons from the literature. *Nursing Times* 114 (5): 34–37.

Harrold, A. (2016). Nurses on the cheap? The nursing associate role examined. www.nursinginpractice.com/professional/training/nurses-on-the-cheap-the-nursing-associate-role-examined

Jones-Berry, S. (2019). The crucial gap in the People Plan's workforce target. *Nursing Standard* 34 (8): 51–53.

King, R., Ryan, T., Wood, E. et al. (2020). Motivations, experiences and aspirations of trainee nursing associates in England: a qualitative study. *BMC Health Services Research* 20: 802.

Lam, P., Lopez Filici, A., Middleton, C., and McGillicuddy, P. (2018). Exploring healthcare professionals' perceptions of the anesthesia assistant role and its impact on patients and interprofessional collaboration. *Journal of Interprofessional Care* 32 (1): 24–32.

Lauder, W. and Roxburgh, M. (2006). Editorial: are there lessons to be learned by the demise of enrolled nurse training in the United Kingdom? *Nurse Education in Practice* 6: 61–62.

Lucas, G., Daniel, D., Thomas, T. et al. (2021). Healthcare professionals' perspectives on enrolled nurses, practical nurses and other second-level roles: a systematic review and thematic synthesis. *International Journal of Nursing Studies* 115: 103844.

McGough, G. and McGough, S. (1998). Enrolled nursing: evaluating the role. *Nursing Standard* 12 (33): 49–56.

NHS (n.d.). Nursing associate. www.healthcareers.nhs.uk/explore-roles/nursing/roles-nursing/nursing-associate

NHS Digital (2024). NHS Vacancy Statistics England, April 2015 – December 2023, Experimental Statistics. https://digital.nhs.uk/data-and-information/publications/statistical/nhs-vacancies-survey/april-2015---december-2023-experimental-statistics

Nursing and Midwifery Council (NMC) (2019). Major milestone reached as first registered nursing associates join health and care workforce. www.nmc.org.uk/news/press-releases/major-milestone-reached-as-first-registered-nursing-associates-join-health-and-care-workforce

Nursing and Midwifery Council (NMC) (2023). The NMC register England mid-year update 1 April – 30 September 2023. www.nmc.org.uk/globalassets/sitedocuments/data-reports/sep-2023/0130b-mid-year-data-report-england-web.pdf

Schindel, T.J., Yuksel, N., Breault, R. et al. (2017). Perceptions of pharmacists' roles in the era of expanding scopes of practice. *Research in Social Administrative Pharmacy* 13 (1): 148–161.

Seccombe, I., Smith, G., Buchan, J. and Ball, J. (1997). Enrolled Nurses: A Study for the UKCC. www.employment-studies.co.uk/system/files/resources/files/344.pdf

Statutory Instrument (1983). The Nurses, Midwives and Health Visitors Rule Approval Order 1983. SI No 873. www.legislation.gov.uk/uksi/1983/873/pdfs/uksi_19830873_en.pdf

Thomas, K. (2016). The NHS is desperately short of nurses. Could a new role hold the answer? www.theguardian.com/healthcare-network/2016/feb/24/nursing-workforce-vacancies-nhs-nurse-associates

Willis, G.P. (2015). *Raising the Bar. Shape of Caring: A Review of the Future Education and Training of Registered Nurses and Care Assistants*. London: Health Education England.

3 Being a Professional: The Importance of Scope of Practice

Claire Agnew van Asch

University Hospitals of Leicester NHS Trust, Leicester, England

Introduction

This chapter explores the importance of transitioning to a registered role and the influence of professionalism within this role. As an NA, you will be expected to uphold the personal and professional standards required by your regulatory body, the Nursing and Midwifery Council (NMC). You will reflect on your development and consider what being a professional means to you in both your personal life and your day-to-day practice, and your engagement with others in the nursing and wider healthcare teams.

This chapter will focus on the importance of understanding your scope of practice and how this relates to your decision making and critical thinking in ensuring that you are providing evidence-based nursing care. Core concepts will be identified which will be developed further in subsequent chapters. Throughout this chapter, the term 'nursing' includes the nursing associate role.

Aims of This Chapter

This chapter will support you to:

- develop your awareness of professional practice
- reflect on key concepts including 'being a professional', advocacy, empathy, autonomy and working within your scope of practice
- consider the importance of clinical decision making, critical thinking and evidence-based practice
- explore some of the fundamental tools to support your practice such as the importance of an effective nurse–patient relationship in providing safe, effective, person-centred care.

The Nursing Associate: Stepping into Practice, First Edition. Edited by Annabel Coulson.
© 2025 John Wiley & Sons Ltd. Published 2025 by John Wiley & Sons Ltd.

- *Platform 1 Being an Accountable Professional.*
- *Platform 3.7 Demonstrate and Apply an Understanding of How and When to Escalate to the Appropriate Professional for Expert Help and Advice.*

Being a Professional

Modern Nursing Origins

Understanding the origins of modern nursing and what is currently influencing its future development will help you make sense of your new professional role and how it fits into the nursing world. Nursing as we know it today started to emerge in the 1850s when advances in modern medicine enabled a leap in its development. Think of nursing and the name that usually springs to mind is Florence Nightingale and the positive impact she had on the health and wellbeing of soldiers in the Crimean War through improvements in general conditions and cleanliness. More recently, Mary Seacole has also been recognised for her role in the Crimean war in setting up a convalescence home for those wounded on the battlefield. Both Florence Nightingale and Mary Seacole are recognised as pioneering nurses who started to shape the profession we have today.

For more information on Florence Nightingale and Mary Seacole please see:

www.florence-nightingale.co.uk/florence-nightingale-biography

www.florence-nightingale.co.uk/mary-seacole

Defining a 'Profession'

> *Any type of work that needs special training or a particular skill, often one that is respected because it involves a high level of education*
>
> *(Cambridge Dictionary 2025)*

Nursing has traditionally been regarded as a vocation in providing services to others. This may be due to the early roots of nursing being linked with religious orders and reflects Florence Nightingale's belief that nursing was a calling. By the second half of the twentieth century, nursing across the globe was striving for professional status to acknowledge the complexities and demands of the role. Table 3.1 compares nursing alongside the well-documented characteristics of a profession (Greenwood 1957; Keogh 1997).

Professional Regulation

The Nurses Registration Act 1919 established the requirement for a statutory register to be kept listing qualified nurses who had met a standard of training and examinations. The NMC is the regulatory body with this responsibility for

Table 3.1: Characteristics of a profession.

Characteristics of a profession	Applied to nursing
It has a theoretical body of specialist knowledge and extended practical training	There is a global specialist body of knowledge specifically for nursing and criteria-led training
It provides a specific service	Yes, nursing is a social service
It has its own professional organisation and is self-regulating	Yes, nursing associates must register with the NMC to practise legally
It requires continuous professional development of its members	Yes, nursing associates are required to demonstrate continuous professional development through revalidation
It has a code of ethics for practice	Yes, nursing associates are required to adhere to the NMC Code
Its members have autonomy in decision making and practice	Yes, the NMC code requires accountability and autonomy to practise

nursing associates. The NMC was formed through the Nursing and Midwifery Order 2001 and its role is to protect the public by:

- maintaining a register of nurses, nursing associates, midwives and health visitors licensed to practise in the UK
- setting standards of education, training, conduct and performance
- ensuring nurses, midwives and health visitors keep their skills and knowledge up to date through revalidation and uphold professional standards set out in the Code
- investigate nurses and midwives who fall short of the standards in the Code (www.nmc.org.uk/about–us/our–role).

Nursing Associate Registered is a title protected by law and it is illegal for someone to use that title if they are not on the NMC register (www.nmc.org.uk/registration/your–registration/legal–basis–of–registration).

Anyone can search the register. The register is public and a live document. If you are now registered, try searching for yourself on the public register to see what can be seen about you.

The NMC Code (NMC 2018b) is the document that steers your professional life and sets out the expectations of professional behaviours, values, accountability and standards of practice of nursing associates, nurses and midwives. The professionalism of nurses and midwives has always been essential to good care. We all know professionalism when we see it but there has never been a single definition for what it means in nursing and midwifery. The 'Enabling professionalism in nursing and midwifery practice' document (NMC 2016) sets out what professionalism looks like in everyday practice through the application of the Code and will help you to reflect on your own practice.

The NMC has also provided a range of videos to illustrate the Code in action called 'Caring with Confidence'. The topics include accountability, professional judgement, delegation, speaking up and professionalism. They can be viewed here: www.nmc.org.uk/standards/code/code–in–action

> **Reflective Activity**
>
> While watching these videos, reflect on what they mean to you as a registered nursing associate and how you can embed the Code into your practice.

Being a Nursing Associate

The sections in this part of the chapter will get you thinking about some of the skills you need to develop your professional self, including advocacy, empathy, autonomy and working within scope, professional judgement and clinical decision making, critical thinking and using the evidence.

Advocacy

Most people can speak up for themselves but put them into unfamiliar and stressful situations, or ones where they feel out of control, and they may not be able to. Have you ever been in a situation where after the event you think 'I wish I had said/done/asked that instead'?

> **Reflective Activity**
>
> Take a moment to think what advocacy means to you.

Advocacy: speaking or acting on behalf of another, supporting and enabling them to:

- express their views and concerns
- access information and services
- defend and promote their rights and responsibilities
- explore choices and options (Bu and Jezewski 2007; Choi 2015).

Patients' rights and expectations are clearly explained in the NHS Constitution, published in 2012 (updated in 2023), available at www.gov.uk/government/publications/the-nhs-constitution-for-england/the-nhs-constitution-for-england.

Patient advocacy is not merely the defence of infringements of patient rights. One of the basic foundations of advocacy in nursing is the patient's right to make decisions that affect their health, particularly for those who may be considered vulnerable in society because of factors such as illness, capacity, culture or equality. Your role is to provide information that helps a patient make decisions and to speak up for them as necessary. You should support an alert, competent patient even if they make decisions that seem unreasonable or harmful, such as the patient who refuses their medications or chooses not to have a particular treatment. This may mean taking a position that may conflict with everyone else, so good communication skills, tact and honesty are important to enable you to advocate effectively.

There are many statements in the NMC Code that support your role of being an advocate for your patients but 3.4 in section 3 specifically mentions the role.

3 Make sure that people's physical, social and psychological needs are assessed and responded to. To achieve this, you must:

> 3.4 *act as an advocate for the vulnerable, challenging poor practice and discriminatory attitudes and behaviour relating to their care.*

Reflective Activity

Take a moment to think about advocacy and how you will support a patient to promote their own wellbeing, as understood by them, and act on their behalf, placing them at the centre of their care.

Barriers to Effective Advocacy

You may experience barriers to being an effective advocate for your patients. It can be very uncomfortable to be a lone voice that is not listened to when you are trying to do the best for your patients. Some reasons for this may be as follows.

- *Powerlessness/helplessness*: feeling like you cannot speak out due to clash of personalities, culture of your clinical area or having self-doubt – you have spoken up before and nothing has been done.
- *Lack of support*: if you are not supported to do your job well, can you be an effective advocate for your patients? What will you do if no one will stand beside you?
- *Medical dominance*: the perception that the doctor is in charge and not to be challenged.
- *Time constraints*: lack of time to get to know your patients so you have a clear picture of their beliefs and wishes, such as when there are staff shortages or appointments are time limited. Also having to make decisions within a short space of time or in an emergency.
- *Loyalty to the team*: the 'we are all in this together' mentality and 'I don't want to drop my colleagues in it' is a particular challenge if you are new to the team and are trying to fit in and establish working relationships.
- *Communication challenges*: caring for a diverse population and people who may not be able to make their needs known.

Advocacy Skills

What skills do you need to be an advocate for your patient? Your role is to build rapport with those you are caring for so you can advocate effectively for them. Some of the following skills will help you do that.

- *Listening*: taking time to listen in confidence; this is not about keeping secrets or colluding with the patient but actively listening and ensuring that they feel they have truly been heard (see section on active listening later in this chapter).

- *Empathy*: have genuine interest in the person, supporting them with honesty and integrity – empathy is discussed in more detail below.
- *Knowing the system*: having knowledge of people's rights and entitlements, local services and procedures. This video by the King's Fund demonstrates the complexities of navigating the care system (www.kingsfund.org.uk/insight-and-analysis/animations/how-does-nhs-england-work). Supporting patients to speak to the right people to get help and advice is a key role of an advocate through 'knowing someone who can...'. The King's Fund also produce some useful 'in a nutshell' information and data to help people understand the NHS, health, and social care in England which you may find helpful (www.kingsfund.org.uk/insight-and-analysis/projects/nhs-in-nutshell).
- *Negotiation skills*: being assertive but not aggressive, having excellent communication skills with tact and diplomacy to get what you need for your patient.
- *Tenacity*: being persistent, trying all available options; there is always someone to ask, and you should not be afraid to escalate your concerns if you feel that you are not being listened to.
- *Independence*: being free from conflict of interest, not swayed by others, not giving in to peer pressure or taking the 'easier path'.

Reflective Activity

Consider the following hypothetical scenarios – what would you do to advocate for the patient? Think about how you will remain person centred and what you may need to do to help refine your advocacy skills to meet the responsibilities set out in the NMC Code.

Scenario 1   Your patient has just had surgery. She has had her pain medicine but an hour later she is still in a lot of pain. The medicine prescription chart shows she can't have another dose for three more hours.

Scenario 2   You are doing a routine check-up for one of your patients at your GP surgery. They confide in you that they are confused about a recent appointment with their GP who mentioned a scan to see if they have 'something nasty' on their chest.

Scenario 3   It is very important to your patient in maintaining his religious beliefs that he prays at certain times every day. However, a procedure off the ward has been scheduled during prayer time the next day.

Scenario 4   A new mother is critically ill following a haemorrhage after birth. She is in ITU and desperately wants to see her baby in case she dies. But infants are not allowed into ITU and the mother can't be moved.

Scenario 5   During a home visit with one of your regular patients, you find several family members there who seem to be having an argument, and the patient is getting upset.

Scenario 6   You are helping with the distribution of patient meals at lunchtime and a patient who is a strict vegan has been served a plate with meat on it.

Suggested answers are given at the end of this chapter.

Empathy

Empathy is described as the capacity to understand or feel what another person is experiencing. Empathy allows you to see things from the other person's perspective.

> **Reflective Activity**
>
> Take 10 minutes to think about when you have displayed empathy towards your patients/clients – how did you demonstrate this? Also think about when someone may have shown you empathy – how did this make you feel?

The concept of empathy was first pioneered by American psychologist Carl Rogers as a key interpersonal skill central to humanistic and person-centred practices in health and social care (Rogers 1961). Demonstrating empathy demands high-level skills of health professionals, who must not only recognise when it is required but also communicate it to patients. Professional self-awareness is key to being able to develop your skills in empathy and use this important communication skill to build rapport with another person, whether they are a patient, client, colleague or other healthcare professional.

Empathy is often described as 'putting yourself in someone else's shoes' (Jones 2019) but in supporting others, it is important to protect yourself from overidentification with their needs – your aim is to help them rather than feel overwhelmed with their problems. An alternative way to think about this is 'put yourself in someone else's shoes but keep your own socks on'. Doing this provides you with some self-protection and objectivity to help prevent you from becoming overwhelmed with your own feelings, beliefs and values and losing sight of the other person's needs. This should help to avoid the risks of compassion fatigue or burnout. These links provide some further information and support on this.

- www.mind.org.uk/information-support/types-of-mental-health-problems/stress/managing-stress-and-building-resilience
- www.nhs.uk/every-mind-matters/mental-wellbeing-tips/self-help-cbt-techniques/bouncing-back-from-lifes-challenges

Active Listening

Active listening is an interactive process between you and the patient where you are fully concentrating on what is being said rather than just passively 'hearing' the message of the speaker. It will help you to develop your empathy skills as you will need to fully attend to the other person to hear what they are saying; along with using all your senses to pick up additional clues from the person you are communicating with, which could be patients, relatives, carers, co-workers ... anyone!

Barriers to active listening might include the setting, timing of the communication and anxiety about what is going to be said on both sides. It is important to be 'present' for the other person; someone skilled in active listening can make a person feel like they have spent an hour with them when they have spent 10 minutes; it is the quality of the interaction that has this impact, not the quantity of time.

Reflective Activity

How do people know you are actively listening to them? What signs do you give? Write these down and then compare your list to that in Table 3.2. Also consider any specific needs of the people and patients you care for.

Table 3.2: Non-verbal and verbal signs of active listening.

Non-verbal signs of active listening	
Smile	Combined with nods of the head, smiles can be powerful in affirming that messages are being listened to and understood. Be mindful that a smile needs to be appropriate to the situation; it can be encouraging or off-putting depending on the subject being discussed.
Eye contact	It is normal and usually encouraging for the listener to look at the speaker. However, a direct stare can be intimidating so think about how much eye contact is appropriate for the situation.
Posture	An open posture helps provide positive signals that you are actively listening, such as leaning slightly forward, arms resting in a neutral position, slight tilt of the head.
Mirroring	Mirroring the non-verbal signs of the speaker provides reinforcement that you are listening and can help show empathy in more emotional situations.
Not being distracted	Avoid fidgeting or looking distracted such as clock watching, constant looking away at other things, doodling, fiddling with hair; a stillness demonstrates you are focused on the person you are speaking to.
Verbal signs of active listening	
Positive reinforcement	While some positive words of encouragement can be helpful, if overused they can be irritating, patronising and interrupt the flow of the speaker. Use informal verbal signals such as 'yes', 'mmm', 'uh-hu', 'good' sparingly and appropriately.
Remembering	Remembering a few key points and the speaker's name can reinforce that their messages have been received and understood. It can also help with clarification (see below). During longer conversations it may be appropriate to jot down some notes to refer to when questioning or clarifying later.
Questioning	Asking relevant questions and/or making statements that build or help to clarify what the speaker has said shows you have been actively listening and also reinforces that you are interested in what the speaker is saying.

Table 3.2: (Continued)

Verbal signs of active listening	
Reflection	Reflecting to the speaker what they have said, through paraphrasing or exactly repeating their words, helps you to confirm your understanding of what they have said and reinforce what you have heard.
Clarification	Asking relevant questions during your exchange helps you to clarify what you have heard and ensure you are correct in your interpretation of their messages. Using open questions prompts the speaker to expand on things you are not clear about.
Summarising	Providing a summary of what you have heard in your own words allows the speaker to confirm that you have picked up the main points of your discussion and clarify anything you may not have heard correctly. It also helps signal the end of your interaction.

Professional Autonomy and Working within Your Scope of Practice

Being a NA enables you to make discretionary and autonomous decisions based on comprehensive knowledge, clinical expertise and evidence-based findings. Professional autonomy means having the authority to make decisions and the freedom to act in accordance with your professional knowledge base (Skår 2009), using this in a critical manner to provide safe, quality healthcare to patients.

There is a clear link between accountability and autonomy: if you want to be autonomous, you need to take responsibility for your decisions and the results of your actions. However, individual levels of autonomy will vary depending on legislative, organisational and individual factors which is why it is important to know you are working within your scope of practice.

What Is Scope of Practice?

The scope of practice is the range of roles, functions, responsibilities and activities which a registered professional is educated, competent and has authority to perform. Your scope is influenced by the clinical context, the patient's needs, your competence, and your organisation's policies and guidelines. Scope of practice cannot be defined as a simple list of tasks or procedures; healthcare evolves rapidly and professionals must be able to incorporate new knowledge and skills into their practice so a list of 'approved activities' would become out of date very quickly. Scope of practice decisions should be based on the principle that the limits of practice must be determined by the *knowledge and skills* required for *safe and competent* performance, and that the NA is *accountable* for whatever they decide to do or not do.

Your scope of practice is driven by the NMC Code (2018a) and the NMC Standards of Proficiency for Nursing Associates (2018b) from your point of registration; it is important to note that your scope of practice is dynamic – that is, it will change and grow as you progress in your career, and gain postregistration experience and qualifications.

Which parts of the NMC Code apply to scope of practice?

Practise Effectively

6 Always practise in line with the best available evidence. To achieve this, you must:

6.1 make sure that any information or advice given is evidence based, including information relating to using any healthcare products or services

6.2 maintain the knowledge and skills you need for safe and effective practice.

Preserve Safety

13 Recognise and work within the limits of your competence.

The NMC also requires you to 'have an appropriate indemnity arrangement in place relevant to your scope of practice which provides appropriate cover for any practice you take on as a nurse, midwife or nursing associate in the United Kingdom' (12.1 of the NMC Code). See www.nmc.org.uk/registration/joining-the-register/professional-indemnity-arrangement for more information on how you meet this requirement.

Ensuring You Are within Scope of Practice

When considering scope of practice, you need to think about your accountability, autonomy, competence, level of supervision, knowledge and appropriate delegation. Working within your scope of practice is determined by the knowledge and skills you require to be safe and competent. It is also influenced by government legislation or directives, employers' policies and guidelines, changing public expectations and changes in the practice of other health professionals. Your scope should be aligned to your job description and contract of employment.

To support your decisions about scope of practice, focus on the rights, needs, and overall benefit to the patient to enable you to always promote and maintain the highest standards of quality care. Ask yourself these questions.

- Is the task or activity in your job description and contract of employment?
- Do you have the necessary knowledge and training?
- Have you had an assessment of competence, if required?
- Are you covered to do this by your organisation's policies or guidelines?
- Is it in the patient's best interests that you do this?
- Do you feel confident, competent and have up-to-date knowledge to do the task or activity?

There is always someone to ask if you are ever unsure; you must not feel pressured to do something that you feel is outside your scope or competence, and make sure you document your decisions and any conversations.

To help with understanding roles, responsibilities and scope, the NMC has issued a comparison table of the standards of proficiencies for registered nurses and registered nursing associates, identifying the differences between the two roles – you can view this at: www.nmc.org.uk/news/news-and-updates/blog-whats-a-nursing-associate/

Clinical Competence

You need a good understanding of clinical competence to work within your scope of practice. A useful model to help you assess your level of clinical competence is Benner's Stages of Clinical Competence (Benner 1984). This model provides a structure of decision making that demonstrates the increase in levels of autonomy, intuition and expertise as a professional develops from novice to expert practice. The five stages of clinical competence highlight that expertise is a process learned over time. You can move both up and down this model; for example, if you change roles, move to an unfamiliar specialty or take on more responsibility, you may temporarily move back down the stages while you gain new knowledge and expertise.

Professional Judgement and Clinical Decision Making

'Judgement' – The ability to make considered decisions or to arrive at reasonable conclusions or opinions on the basis of the available information
(Oxford English Dictionary 2013)

Professional judgements inform clinical decisions, and the terms are frequently used interchangeably along with clinical judgement and clinical reasoning. The process of exercising judgement or making decisions can often be an almost unconscious activity; but for complex and challenging decisions it is important that you are consciously aware of the decision you need to make, and can do so objectively and analytically. Professional self-awareness and reflective practice will support the ongoing development of your professional judgement and clinical decision-making skills.

The process of professional judgement involves using different aspects of information (which may be about a person, object or situation) to arrive at an overall evaluation. In nursing, this could be considered as the process of using different types of clinical information about the patient (such as appearance, vital signs, and behaviour) to assess their current health status.

There are several factors that frame and inform professional judgement and one way of looking at this is the 'Four Professional Judgment Building Blocks' which can support your decision making

- *Knowledge* – having a professional body of knowledge and specialist training, analysing and using the evidence.
- *Professional obligations* – NMC code and standards of proficiency that drive everything that you do.
- *Patient/client input* – patient choice, expert patient, respecting rights of the individual versus the challenge of best interest.
- *Experience* – including practical wisdom, reflective practice and intuition.

Clinical Decision Making

Judgements feed into decision making in that the assessments or evaluations you make can be used to make choices about nursing care needs. For example, you may assess a patient as being at risk of developing a pressure ulcer (judgement) and then choose a particular intervention to reduce that risk (decision) based on the assessment. The nursing process (see later in the chapter) is a structured framework that can support your decision making. Remember – you will be working with oversight from a registered nurse, so it is important to establish where your professional judgement and decision-making boundaries are in relation to theirs to help you work as an effective team.

The types of decisions you make may include the following.

- How you will organise your workload.
- Prioritisation of care.
- Delegation – what and to whom.
- Making referrals.
- Use of risk assessment tools.
- The need for further information.
- What to communicate and to whom.
- Information on treatment, intervention, health promotion.
- When to escalate care concerns.

Reflective Activity

Is there anything else you can add to this list that relates to your practice area?

The well-known '5WH' question model can help gather information to enable you to make clinical decisions.

- *What*: the problem is.
- *Why*: is it a problem and why now?
- *Who*: is it a problem for?
- *When and Where*: is it a problem?
- How: can the problem be addressed?

Complex decision making requires an objective and analytical approach and should not be made in isolation without additional guidance and support. You can get further information, advice and support from the following.

- Your organisation's policies and guidelines.
- Ethical frameworks.
- The NMC Code.
- Available evidence of best practice such as National Institute of Health and Care excellence (NICE) guidance.
- Your experience, knowledge and skills base.
- Experience and views of other healthcare professionals.
- Choice and capacity of your patient/carers.
- Decisions previously made in similar situations.
- Reflection on practice.

The NMC Code has extensive guidance on making professional judgements and clinical decisions, some of the statements are listed below:

2.4 Respect the level to which people receiving care want to be involved in decisions about their own health, wellbeing and care.

6.　Always practise in line with the best available evidence; to achieve this, you must:

   6.1　make sure that any information or advice given is evidence based, including information relating to using any healthcare products or services, and

   6.2　maintain the knowledge and skills you need for safe and effective practice.

9.3　Deal with differences of professional opinion with colleagues by discussion and informed debate, respecting their views and opinions and behaving in a professional way at all times.

20.6　Stay objective and have clear professional boundaries at all times with people in your care (including those who have been in your care in the past), their families and carers.

20.7　Make sure you do not express your personal beliefs (including political, religious or moral beliefs) to people in an inappropriate way.

Critical Thinking and Using the Evidence

Developing your critical thinking skills will help you use tools like the nursing process (see later in the chapter) and apply your professional judgement and make decisions in a systematic and logical way.

Critical thinking requires you to think clearly and rationally, use reason, reflection, and think independently without influence. Critical thinkers are active learners, not passive recipients of information; they rigorously question ideas and assumptions rather than accepting them at face value. They will always seek to understand connections between ideas and findings, determine whether these represent the entire picture, and are open to finding that they may not. Being a critical thinker will help you develop an inquisitive, well-informed, ethical, responsible approach to making nursing decisions and planning nursing care and avoid situations where care is provided as 'this is the way we have always done it' or 'because I said so'.

Critical thinking involves:

- questioning what is usually taken for granted
- reflecting on the reasons for doing things, evaluating values, beliefs and assumptions and asking 'is this justifiable?'
- having curiosity, a healthy scepticism, keeping an open mind
- asking the 5WH questions (see above).

Using Evidence-based Practice

Using evidence-based practice alongside critical thinking will enable you to provide a clear rationale for the care you give and ensure it is up to date and based on the best available evidence. Evidence-based practice recognises that care is individualised and ever changing and involves uncertainties and probabilities. It is traditionally defined in terms of a 'three-legged stool' integrating three basic principles.

- The best available research evidence bearing on whether and why a treatment works – credible evidence, systematic reviews.

- Professional judgement/clinical expertise (clinical judgement and experience) to rapidly identify each patient's unique health state and diagnosis, and the individual risks and benefits of potential interventions.
- Client preferences and values.

Read more about evidence-based practice in Chapter 8.

Foundations for the Nursing Associate Role

This section draws together all the themes discussed so far in this chapter and discusses some of the foundations for your practice, focusing on the nurse–patient relationship and the nursing process and how important these are in enabling effective person-centred care.

The Nurse–Patient Relationship

> *The relationship between a nurse and the person in their care is a professional relationship based on trust and respect to meet the person's needs and health outcomes.*
>
> *(Feo et al. 2017)*

Fundamental to a positive nurse–patient relationship is your ability to build rapport, based on open communication, trust, understanding, compassion and kindness. The foundations of all good nurse–patient relationships are built on your ability to listen (with all senses, not just your ears) and respond to the patient as an individual.

> **Reflective Activity**
>
> Consider the following quote. What do you think about this? How do you create a good first impression? What is a good first impression?
> "Nurses are never invisible, nurses are always seen, always noticed and always judged for better or worse." (Radcliffe 2011)

First impressions may include judgements about you by the patient and/or their relatives and carers such as whether you introduce yourself and ask the patient their preferred name, have a welcoming and friendly approach, whether your mode of dress is clean and tidy and conveys a professional image? Do you look rushed and harassed? Do you seem to know what you are doing? Is your working environment in control or chaos? These first impressions will impact on your ability to effectively build rapport and trust.

The Ipsos MORI Veracity Index is an annual index of which jobs and professionals are most trusted by the public; this poll has been conducted consistently since 1983, making it the longest running series on trust in key professions in the UK. Nurses have been included in the list of professions since 2016 and every year since they have come top. You can see the results for 2024 here: https://www.ipsos.com/en-uk/ipsos-veracity-index-2024

Reflective Activity

How does this level of trust in your profession by the public make you feel?

Requirements for a Successful Nurse–Patient Relationship

- *Positive regard*: an unconditional, non-judgemental attitude.
- *Respect*: regardless of the patient's background, behaviour or lifestyle.
- *Acceptance*: not responding negatively or being upset by a patient's outburst or anger.
- *Genuine interest*: authentic communication.
- *Empathy*.
- *Trust*.
- *Confidentiality*: within the boundaries of the NMC Code.
- *Self-awareness*; developing an understanding of your own values, beliefs, thoughts, feelings, attitudes, motivations, prejudices, strengths and limitations and how these qualities affect others.

You may find that you use many aspects of your personality to build rapport and establish a relationship with your patient such as your previous experiences, values, feelings, emotional intelligence, coping skills, and perceptions. This is why self-awareness is so important as a professional to enable you to draw on all these aspects as part of your nurse–patient relationship while also setting boundaries and managing expectations.

Humour can enable the nurse to 'treat people as individuals' and develop the therapeutic nurse–patient relationship. Humour can appear slightly at odds with the NMC Code which focuses on professional behaviour and practice, but it is a natural expression of emotion and has a place in providing holistic and personalised care when used appropriately (Tremayne 2014).

On the other side of this, you may have difficulty in building rapport; this may be due to a variety of reasons and misjudging a nurse–patient relationship can result in frustration and anger from the patient and a reluctance to communicate with you. Taking a step back to objectively consider what might be behind their outburst, you may find that feelings such as fear, anxiety, confusion, guilt, stress, embarrassment or being overwhelmed could explain what is going on for that person and some of their behaviours.

The NMC Code provides clear expectations of your role in developing a positive nurse–patient relationship:

Prioritise People

> You put the interests of people using or needing nursing or midwifery services first. You make their care and safety your main concern and make sure that their dignity is preserved, and their needs are recognised, assessed and responded to. You make sure that those receiving care are treated with respect, that their rights are upheld and that any discriminatory attitudes and behaviours towards those receiving care are challenged.

Promote Professionalism and Trust

You uphold the reputation of your profession at all times. You should display a personal commitment to the standards of practice and behaviour set out in the Code. You should be a model of integrity and leadership for others to aspire to. This should lead to trust and confidence in the professions from patients, people receiving care, other health and care professionals and the public.

20.6 Stay objective and have clear professional boundaries at all times with people in your care (including those who have been in your care in the past), their families and carers.

Reflective Activity

Take some time to reflect on how you will adhere to the NMC Code as a NA to build your nurse–patient relationships.

How Do You Build a Nurse–Patient Relationship?

The six-stage model of relationship forming (see below) is one example of how you can build a nurse–patient relationship. There is no set timeframe for this – you may go through all these stages within a 10-minute outpatient or GP appointment, during a 12-week course of therapy, such as chemotherapy or rehabilitation, or during an overnight stay in hospital. These phases can also apply to the relationships you build with patients' relatives and carers.

Six-stage Model of Relationship Forming
1. *Contact*: first impressions, social exchange, a greeting.
2. *Involvement*: a sense of connection and mutuality is established; may be questions.
3. *Intimacy*: professional connection through empathy, understanding and closeness.
4. *Deterioration*: preparing for discharge from care; this phase is inevitable.
5. *Repair*: if patient returns to your care at this point, you return to stage 3.
6. *Dissolution*: patient is discharged from your care (DeVito 2022).

Reflective Activity

Use the six-stage model of relationship formation to reflect on your nurse–patient relationship interactions. Think of times when things went well and not so well and consider what skills you employed to build rapport and trust and how these helped or hindered you.

Holistic Nursing Care

You will be able to read more about this in Chapter 4.

Holistic nursing is a philosophy and a model and is based on fundamental theories of nursing, such as the works of Florence Nightingale and more recently Jean Watson's theory of human caring (read more about this here: www. watsoncaringscience.org).

Holistic nursing care:

- sees the patient as a whole – not just a disease or condition
- is an approach or value system held by practitioners who provide care which recognises the patient as a whole person with physical, psychological, sociological and spiritual dimensions
- embraces the mind, body and spirit of the patient in a culture that supports a therapeutic nurse–patient relationship resulting in wholeness, harmony and healing (Baillie and Black 2015, pp.153–154).

Holistic nursing care provides the foundations of a nurse–patient relationship and underpins the ability to build rapport and trust and ensure that the patient remains the focus of all care decisions.

The Unpopular Patient

Seminal work by Stockwell in 1972 examined the term 'the unpopular patient', looking at behaviours and attitudes of patients that may make them unpopular with the nursing staff. This research study investigated the interpersonal relationships between nurses and patients in general hospital wards and challenged the view held at the time that nurses treated all patients in a non-judgemental way.

Four factors were identified as affecting the nurse–patient relationship.

- *Personality factors*: was the patient cheerful, pleasant, selfish, bad-tempered?
- *Communication factors*: was the patient grateful, amusing, uncooperative, grumbling?
- *Attitude factors*: were they understanding, optimistic, unwilling to accept treatment, reluctant to go home?
- *Nursing factors*: were they interesting to nurse, needed nursing, did not need to be in hospital, not well known (Stockwell 1972, pp. 26–27)?

In a nursing context, the implication for unpopular patients is that they may be more likely to be excluded by nursing staff, reinforcing social isolation at a time when they are at their most vulnerable. Patients who feel devalued may experience feelings of insecurity, anguish and failure (Stockwell 1972).

You can find the original publication by searching for 'the unpopular patient' in the patient experience library available at: www.patientlibrary.net/cgi-bin/library.cgi

The Nursing Process

Nursing has been described as:

> *a unique blend of art and science applied within the context of interpersonal relationships for the purpose of promoting wellness, preventing illness and restoring health in individuals, families and communities.*
>
> (Wilkinson 2007, p.1)

The nursing process could be considered where the science of nursing starts to blend with the art of nursing. Think about all the interactions you have with patients, clients, relatives, carers, team members, other healthcare professionals, people outside the healthcare world – consider whether the skills you need to interact and communicate effectively with all these different groups take both an art and science approach with the evidence base supporting the skills you have.

What Is the Nursing Process?

- The nursing process is a problem-solving systematic approach to providing safe, individualised nursing care.
- It was first described as a four-stage process by Ida Jean Orlando in 1958 and became a well-established approach to nursing by the 1970s.

The nursing process could be considered one of the 'tools of the trade'. It enables you to organise your work, systematically consider your actions and solve problems, document the care you provide and measure its outcomes; it supports a systematic way of thinking and acting, and encourages a creative and intuitive approach to care.

The nursing process:

- promotes collaboration
- is cost-effective
- helps people understand what nurses do
- supports professional standards of practice
- increases patient/client participation in care and promotes autonomy
- promotes individualised care
- promotes efficiency
- fosters continuity and co-ordination of care
- increases job satisfaction (Wilkinson 2007, pp.7–9).

When used alongside a nursing model (see Chapter 4), it facilitates consistent, evidence-based nursing care. It is a framework for clinical decision making which helps to guide the planning and delivery of patient care, promotes critical thinking, enhances quality of clinical decision making and promotes professionalism.

It is a cyclical process made up of five components – Assessment, Diagnosis, Planning, Implementing and Evaluating – often abbreviated to ADPIE.

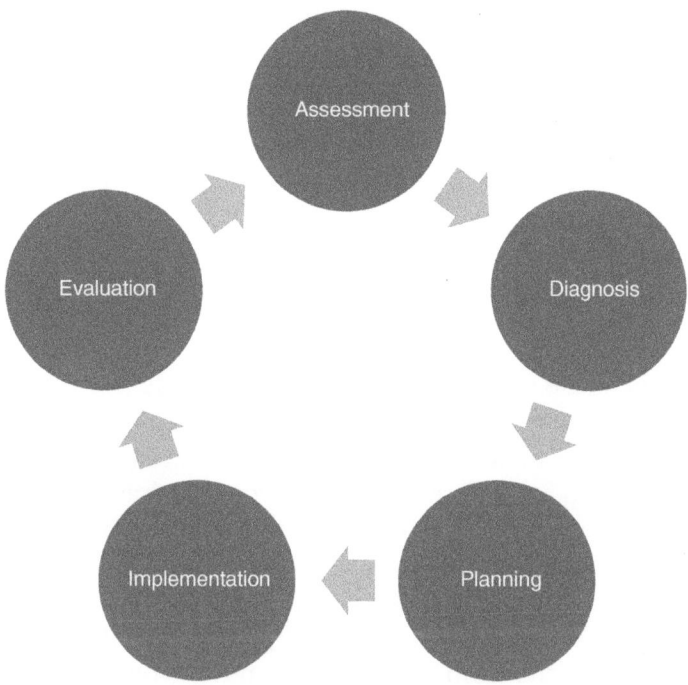

Assessment   In this phase you will complete some assessments, such as obtaining biographical details including name, date of birth, age, address, clinical observations such as blood pressure, pulse and respiration. You may also ask for relevant medical, personal and social history and undertake screening or risk assessments using specific clinical assessment tools such as those for pain or pressure ulcer prevention. Although considered to be the starting point of the nursing process, the assessment phase is ongoing; it is a fundamental skill that is the first step to ensuring holistic and individualised care, gathering information on the psychological, sociocultural, spiritual and environmental needs of your patient as well as medical needs, and assessment of patient problems, concerns and issues.

There is still debate about the NA's role in assessment; currently NAs will not do an 'initial or primary' assessment of the patient. You need to consider the difference between assessment and gathering data to support the RN to complete the 'initial or primary' assessment.

During the assessment you will collect two main types of data.

- *Subjective data* cannot be directly measured or observed, such as opinions, feelings, description of symptoms.
- *Objective data* are measurable and can be seen, heard, felt or smelt. Because objective data are measurable, they are often referred to as signs.

Reflective Activity

Think about all the data you collect on your patients. What tools or methods do you use? How do you know that the information is consistent and valid?

Diagnosis   A nursing diagnosis is about using the social sciences as well as clinical risk assessments and seeing the patient as a whole – holistically! As a NA, your current scope of practice does not enable you to undertake a nursing diagnosis but you can make recommendations to the RN about a plan of care based on the data you collect in the assessment phase. The diagnosis is used to identify the patient's needs or problems and develop outcomes or goal setting to meet these needs in order of priority.

Planning   This phase of the nursing process extends from the assessment and in conjunction with the patient or client, wherever possible, you will agree how the care needs are to be met. You will use your nursing knowledge to put a care plan in place to achieve the care goals you may have set with or for the patient. To do this effectively, you need to work alongside the RN who has overall responsibility for care planning.

Goals may be short term or long term and must focus on the individual and be easily achieved. The care and interventions planned should also be developed and communicated to the team, so everyone knows what you and the patient are aiming to achieve.

Implementing   The implementation phase is the actionable part of the nursing process where you carry out the interventions you have identified; as part of your plan, you will document care and work with other healthcare professionals to meet the needs of the patient. The implementation phase may be performed using a combination of direct care and indirect care.

- *Direct care* is care given directly to the patient in either a physical or verbal manner. It may include assisting the patient with mobility, performing physical interventions and assisting with daily living activities. It may also include coaching, counselling and providing feedback.
- *Indirect care* is care that is given while away from the patient. It may include monitoring or supervising the effects of interventions performed by others, delegating care responsibilities and advocating on behalf of the patient.

You will use your critical thinking and professional judgement skills here to question the care plan to ensure it is meeting the needs of your patient. Steps or procedures that appear to be inappropriate, non-actionable or not achievable should be questioned and re-evaluated.

Evaluating   Evaluations of the effectiveness of the care you have planned should be undertaken frequently and in line with the interventions made. Questions to consider include the following.

- Have the goals planned with the patient been achieved?
- Has the need or problem improved or deteriorated? Was the goal appropriate? Was the nursing care appropriate? Is additional information required?

Evaluation is ongoing and leads directly back to the assessment phase of the nursing process, changing and adapting the care plan accordingly.

Sometimes this process might happen quickly, for example in a cardiac arrest or in an emergency; whereas in health promotion situations such as supporting someone to stop smoking, the process will be more long term.

The nursing process can be both simple and complex in its application and it is only as good as the person using it. Applying it effectively requires a significant amount of skill and understanding to do it well and involves the following skills.

- *Cognitive (intellectual) skills*: decision making and critical thinking, reflection, rational and reasonable thought.
- *Creativity and curiosity*: vision, insight, asking the 5WH questions.
- *Effective interpersonal skills*.
- *Cultural competence*: working within the person's belief system; knowledge of and respect for the cultural values and behaviours of others.
- *Psychomotor skills*: 'hands-on' care.
- *Technological skills* (Wilkinson 2007; Alfaro-Lefevre 2010).

The nursing process is often not talked about directly but it is embedded in practice as a core element of delivering high-quality and considered nursing care as set out in the NMC Code and standards of proficiencies:

Practise Effectively

You assess need and deliver or advise on treatment or give help (including preventative or rehabilitative care) without too much delay, to the best of your abilities, on the basis of best available evidence.

NMC Proficiencies

Nursing associates provide compassionate, safe and effective care and support to people in a range of care settings; you monitor the condition and health needs of people within your care on a continual basis in partnership with people, families and carers. You contribute to ongoing assessment and can recognise when it is necessary to refer to others for reassessment.

Chapter Summary

This chapter has set the scene for your professional practice and examined concepts including being a professional, advocacy, empathy, autonomy and working within scope, professional judgement and clinical decision making, critical thinking and evidence-based practice. It explores some of the fundamental aspects of your practice such as the nurse–patient relationship and how using this alongside the nursing process provides a foundation for safe, effective, person-centred care.

Suggested Answers for Advocacy Scenarios

Scenario 1

Your patient has just had surgery. She has had her pain medicine but an hour later she is still in a lot of pain. The medicine prescription chart shows she can't have another dose for three more hours.

What do you do?

Repeat the pain score, discuss with RN and doctors to get PRN medication or pain relief review, and while waiting for this consider repositioning/distraction therapy. Does the patient have other complementary options such as heat or a TENS machine? Consider contacting the pain specialist nursing team for further support.

Scenario 2

You are doing a routine check-up for one of your patients at your GP surgery. They confide in you that they are confused about a recent appointment with their GP who mentioned a scan to see if they have 'something nasty' on their chest.

What do you do?

The key thing here is to reassure the patient and work within your scope of practice. Maybe ask some more questions to clarify what the patient is thinking and ask them what they would like you to do. Be mindful that despite looking at the notes (if you would usually have access to these), the doctor's conversation may not be clear so it is always best to not try and guess.

If the patient gives consent, you could speak to someone on their behalf. Speak to the practice nurse and GP and feed back the conversation with the patient and request follow-up by the GP who made the comment so they can explain more fully. You could recommend the patient has someone with them for the conversation with the GP to provide support.

Scenario 3

It is very important to your patient in maintaining his religious beliefs that he prays at certain times every day. However, a procedure off the ward has been scheduled during prayer time the next day.

What do you do?

You could contact the department to see if the procedure is time critical or whether there is a possibility to move the time. If the time cannot be changed, check with the patient – would he consider praying at an alternative time? Would he like a visit from the chaplaincy team to help with his decision?

Scenario 4

A new mother is critically ill following a haemorrhage after birth. She is in ITU and desperately wants to see her baby in case she dies. But infants are not allowed into ITU and the mother can't be moved.

What do you do?

Consider whether an exception can be made in this instance – escalate to your senior team for support and advice. While this is being sorted out, continue to seek alternative ways of communicating and connecting mum and baby – can you use a device to Facetime/Zoom, ask for pictures, handprints/footprints to help with memories, provide something of mum's to the baby?

Scenario 5

During a home visit with one of your regular patients, you find several family members there who seem to be having an argument, and the patient is getting upset.

What do you do?

It is important to ask the patient what they want to do and also make sure both you and they are safe. Speak to the family and explain how they are making the patient feel – they may not realise this. State that your patient is your priority and you will ask them to leave if they continue to upset the patient. Get support from other team members if you are working alone. If the situation escalates, you may need to involve the police for immediate safety and wellbeing needs. Consider potential safeguarding issues as well.

Scenario 6

You are helping with the distribution of patient meals at lunchtime and a patient who is a strict vegan has been served a plate with meat on it.

What do you do?

Apologise to the patient and arrange for a suitable meal to be delivered. Try to find out how it had happened, communicate to the rest of the team and document meal requirements to help prevent it from happening again.

References

Alfaro-LeFevre, R. (2010). *Applying Nursing Process. A Tool for Critical Thinking*. Philadelphia: Wolters Kluwer/Lippincott Williams and Wilkins.

Baillie, L. and Black, S. (2015). *Professional Values in Nursing*. Boca Raton: CRC Press.

Benner, P. (1984). *From Novice to Expert: Excellence and Power in Clinical Nursing Practice*. New Jersey: Prentice Hall Health.

Bu, X. and Jezewski, M.A. (2007). Developing a mid-range theory of patient advocacy through concept analysis. *Journal of Advanced Nursing* 57 (1): 101–110.

Cambridge Dictionary. (2025). *Profession. Available at:* https://dictionary.cambridge.org/dictionary/english/profession (Accessed 19 January 2025).

Choi, P.P. (2015). Patient advocacy: the role of the nurse. *Nursing Standard* 29 (41): 52–58.

DeVito, J.A. (2022). *The Interpersonal Communication Book*, 16e. Harlow: Pearson.

Feo, R., Rasmussen, P., Wiechula, R. et al. (2017). Developing effective and caring nurse–patient relationships. *Nursing Standard* 31 (28): 54–63.

Greenwood, E. (1957). Attributes of a profession. *Social Work* 2 (3): 45–55.

Jones, N.P. (2019). The 6Cs. In: *Learning to Care. The Nursing Associate* (ed. I. Peate), 74–82. London: Elsevier.

Keogh, J. (1997). Professionalisation of nursing: development, difficulties and solution. *Journal of Advanced Nursing* 25: 302–308.

Nursing and Midwifery Council (NMC) (2016). *Enabling Professionalism*. London: NMC.

Nursing and Midwifery Council (NMC) (2018b). *Standards of Proficiency for Nursing Associates*. London: Nursing and Midwifery Council.

Nursing and Midwifery Council (NMC) (2018a). *The Code. Professional Standards of Practice and Behaviour for Nurses, Midwives and Nursing Associates*. London: Nursing and Midwifery Council.

Oxford English Dictionary. (2013). *Judgement. Available at:* https://www.oed.com/dictionary/judgement_n?tab=meaning_and_use (Accessed 19 January 2025).

Radcliffe, M. (2011). Opinion: 'Having a smoke with your client used to feel like good nursing'. *Nursing Times* 107: 28.

Rogers, C. (1961). *On Becoming a Person: A Therapist's View of Psychotherapy.* Boston: Houghton Mifflin.

Skår, R. (2009). The meaning of autonomy in nursing practice. *Journal of Clinical Nursing* 19: 2226–2234.

Stockwell, F. (1972). *The Unpopular Patient.* London: Royal College of Nursing.

Tremayne, P. (2014). Using humour to enhance the nurse–patient relationship. *Nursing Standard* 28 (30): 37–40.

Wilkinson, J.M. (2007). *Nursing Process and Critical Thinking*, 4e. New Jersey: Pearson Education Inc.

Further Reading

Alfaro-LeFevre, R. (2020). *Critical Thinking, Clinical Reasoning and Clinical Judgement. A Practical Approach*, 7e. St Louis: Elsevier.

Ali, M. (2018). Communication 5: effective listening and observation skills. *Nursing Times* 114 (4): 60–61.

Buckley, A. and Corless, L. (2016). Patient narratives 5: providing empathetic care in nursing practice. *Nursing Times* 112 (15): 22–23.

Connor, J., Flenady, T., Massey, D., and Dwyer, T. (2022). Clinical judgement in nursing – an evolutionary concept analysis. *Journal of Clinical Nursing* 32 (13–14): 3325–3340.

Ellis, P., Standing, M., Roberts, S., and Howatson-Jones, L. (2020). *Patient Assessment and Care Planning in Nursing*, 3e. London: Sage.

Gillespie, M. and Peterson, B.L. (2009). Helping novice nurses make effective clinical decisions: the situated clinical decision-making framework. *Nursing Education Perspectives* 30 (3): 164–170.

Grant, A. and Goodman, B. (2019). *Communication and Interpersonal Skills in Nursing*, 4e. London: Sage.

Holme, A. (2015). Big ideas: why history matters to nursing. *Nurse Education Today* 35: 635–637.

Nightingale, F. (2015). *Notes on Nursing – What It Is and Is Not* (originally published 1859). CreateSpace independent publishing platform.

Pratt, H., Moroney, T., and Middleton, R. (2021). The influence of engaging authentically on nurse-patient relationships: a scoping review. *Nursing Inquiry* 28: E12388.

Pursio, K., Kankkunen, P., Sanner-Stiehr, E., and Kvist, T. (2021). Professional autonomy in nursing: an integrative review. *Journal of Nursing Management* 29: 1565–1577.

Reed, A. and Dix, A. (2018). A framework to promote professionalism in everyday practice. *Nursing Times* 114 (3): 40–42.

Schmidt, B.J. and McArthur, E.C. (2018). Professional nursing values: a concept analysis. *Nursing Forum* 53: 69–75.

Smith, L. and Mee, S. (2017). Patient advocacy: breaking down barriers and challenging decisions. *Nursing Times* 113 (1): 54–56.

Standing, M. (2017). *Clinical Judgement and Decision Making in Nursing*, 3e. London: Sage.

ten Hoeve, Y., Jansen, G., and Roodbol, P. (2014). The nursing profession: public image, self-concept and professional identity. A discussion paper. *Journal of Advanced Nursing* 70 (2): 295–309.

Wiechula, R., Conroy, T., Kitson, A. et al. (2016). Umbrella review of the evidence: what factors influence the caring relationship between a nurse and a patient. *Journal of Advanced Nursing* 72 (4): 723–734.

4 Applying Person-centred Approaches to Care

Leigh-Ann Cowell

University Hospitals of Leicester NHS Trust, Leicester, UK

Introduction

The nursing associate (NA) role offers healthcare delivery an excellent opportunity to develop a person-centred approach to care planning and delivery. This chapter will explore the role in relation to establishing an early relationship with individuals and sustaining it during the episode of care. Registered nursing associates will be able to explore different approaches to ensuring a person-centred approach while establishing their role in aspects such as admission and assessment and supporting the development of patient-focused care planning.

Aims of This Chapter

- Discuss the ways in which the concepts of choice, autonomy, empowerment, respect, and holism, empathy and compassion should inform and dictate nursing practice.
- Demonstrate the knowledge, communication and relationship skills to deliver person-centred care, considering the wellbeing of the individual, family and carers.
- Explain the importance of working with people to encourage shared decision making and increase independence.
- Describe the role of the nursing associate in the delivery of person-centred care, ensuring that individuals' needs for safety, dignity, privacy, comfort and sleep are met.
- Demonstrate an understanding of how to deliver a person-centred approach to people and their families towards the end of life.
- Explain how the concept of parity of esteem is reflected and enacted in relation to a person-centred approach to care, including the importance of early years and childhood experiences.

The Nursing Associate: Stepping into Practice, First Edition. Edited by Annabel Coulson.
© 2025 John Wiley & Sons Ltd. Published 2025 by John Wiley & Sons Ltd.

Related NMC Standards

- 1.11 Provide, promote and where appropriate advocate for non-discriminatory, person-centred and sensitive care at all times. Reflect on people's values and beliefs, diverse backgrounds, cultural characteristics, language requirements, needs and preferences, taking account of any need for adjustments.
- 2.5 Understand the importance of early years and childhood experiences and the possible impact on life choices, mental, physical and behavioural health and wellbeing.
- 3.4 Demonstrate the knowledge, communication and relationship management skills required to provide people, families and carers with accurate information that meets their needs before, during and after a range of interventions.
- 3.5 Work in partnership with people to encourage shared decision making, in order to support individuals, their families and carers to manage their own care when appropriate.
- 3.8 Demonstrate and apply an understanding of how people's needs for safety, dignity, privacy, comfort and sleep can be met.
- 3.13 Demonstrate an understanding of how to deliver sensitive and compassionate end-of-life care to support people to plan for their end of life, giving information and support to people who are dying, their families and the bereaved. Provide care to the deceased.
- 3.14 Understand and act in line with any end-of-life decisions and orders, organ and tissue donation protocols, infection protocols, advanced planning decisions, living wills and lasting powers of attorney for health.
- 3.23 Recognise people at risk of abuse, self-harm and/or suicidal ideation and the situations that may put them and others at risk.

What Is Person-centred Care?

Person-centred care was a notion developed in the 1970s with the aim of moving away from the patient being defined by a medical subject or problem and towards a model of care that encompasses the needs, wants and goals personally held by the patient (Smith and Willis 2020). There has been a long-standing importance placed on this concept within the nursing profession (McCormack and McCance 2016, p. 1), and the public should be able to trust that they will be treated as individuals, have their human rights respected, be given choices, and supported to make their own decisions regarding their care.

Florence Nightingale is widely recognised as the main influence in establishing modern nursing, and although she may not have specifically used the term 'person-centred care', the focus of her life's work was on the 'person' being cared for, while providing the most conducive environment for healing. So why is there such an emphasis now on developing a person-centred workforce if it is what we should have been doing all along?

Reflective Activity

Think about your last working day. Did you spend time considering how to meet the individual needs of your patients or service users? How did you prioritise your workload? Was it needs based or task based? Did you provide your patients or service users with choices? If so, what were those choices? Would you consider the care you provided to be person centred?

Person-centred care is now the focus of policy and legislation. Several papers discuss the need to develop a more engaged relationship with patients, carers and communities so that we can promote wellbeing and prevent ill health (NHS England 2014; NHS 2019).

To ensure that care is person centred, it must be relevant to the individual, including all the factors that may impact on their care and treatment. To do this, the NA needs to understand the needs of their patient and, together with the registered nurse (RN), be able to agree realistic treatment goals. Once these goals have been established, there can be an agreement on the types of treatment and support services that will be most appropriate to assist in achieving them. When care plans are developed by the RN, the NA needs to ensure that they reflect these needs and preferences.

Person-centred care needs to be co-ordinated; people should not be continually repeating themselves to different professionals so there needs to be a more joined-up approach across health and social care.

Reflective Activity

Think about how you get to know your patients, clients, service users. What matters to them? How are you able to advocate for them to ensure that their needs are met: What challenges will you face with this?

Person-centred care is more than a concept, it is an expectation. Person-centred care is not about being in a specific role or having a level of seniority; it requires the right skills to have meaningful conversations with people and carers using services – we will look later at a range of tools designed to help you with this. The Nursing and Midwifery Council (NMC) (2018) stipulates that NAs should act in the best interests of those they care for, putting them first and delivering care that is person centred, compassionate and safe. The challenge arises when NAs are managing heavy workloads and it becomes more difficult to ensure that true person-centredness is at the heart of their care, all the time.

While you can characterise patients into groups such as age, gender, ethnicity or even diagnosis, we must always remember that every person is a unique individual; for example, while identical twins share many of the same characteristics, their needs, wants, goals and choices make them different from each other (Harris 2021, p. 15).

This personalised approach to care delivery aims to ensure that the choices a person has regarding their treatment will provide them with care appropriate to their specific requirements, leading to positive health outcomes (Hardy 2015).

Many people are no longer content to be cared for, to passively receive treatment while assuming that healthcare professionals 'know best'; many now want to be assisted to help themselves, to learn more about their diagnosis and treatments on offer, to be involved in decisions about their treatments and to potentially seek alternatives that meet their needs, becoming the expert patient (Peate 2019; Harris 2021).

An ever-growing older population demonstrates that people are living longer with long-term conditions and disabilities, thanks to advances in treatments and medication, and person-centred care supports these people to make informed decisions to effectively manage their own health (Health Foundation 2016).

There is no single agreed definition of person-centred care. To be truly person centred, all aspects of care and support need to be moulded to fit the individual, and would support their values, beliefs and choice, and this is why it is difficult to provide a set definition.

Health Foundation (2016) Four Key Principles

- Affording people dignity, compassion, and respect.
- Offering co-ordinated care, support or treatment.
- Offering personalised care, support or treatment.
- Supporting people to recognise and develop their own strengths and abilities, enabling them to live an independent and fulfilling life.

Any care that a person receives should be undertaken with these principles in mind, because any experience that is person centred will include a combination or all of them.

If you consider your role as positioned between the RN and the healthcare assistant (HCA), then you are perfectly placed to support the implementation of core values of nursing, known as the Six Cs (DoH 2021) in the provision of person-centred care. When delivering personal intimate care such as washing, dressing, support with food and nutrition, etc., or less intimate care such as drug administration, collecting information for admission, etc., you have the ideal opportunity to talk to your patient and gain an understanding of their likes and dislikes. You will start to understand how you need to communicate with them and spot non-verbal cues that will tell you more about how they might be feeling.

You need to be clear that this is not a 'HCA' job – you are no longer just washing a patient, you are looking at skin integrity, predicting their needs based on the evidence you are seeing and what you are gleaning from their communication. Explore the roles you have deemed to be 'HCA' roles and look at how you need to approach this differently with the different knowledge and skills you are gaining.

You should be able to develop effective relationships with individuals and families. They may take time to build up but you also have the knowledge to provide evidence-based care and signpost individuals to relevant services and specialists who will be able to provide ongoing specialist support.

The role of the NA in delivering high standards of person-centred care includes moving away from task-orientated care and being an advocate for every individual; understanding the theory behind why you are doing things;

seeking confirmation and support when you do not know something; and identifying when things go wrong and having the courage to raise concerns.

While this approach to healthcare may seem to be common sense, there is a plethora of evidence that suggests it is not common practice, and inquiries into failings in care support this notion, such as those at Mid-Staffordshire and Morecambe Bay hospitals and within social care settings like Winterbourne View (Francis 2013; Kirkup 2015; Hardy 2015).

The NA can use many approaches to support the delivery of person-centred care including nursing theory, nursing models, the nursing process, active listening and effective communication skills.

Nursing Theories and Models

Nursing theories relate to the organisation of knowledge and explanation of what happens in nursing, at a concrete and specific level. 'Nursing theory' is the term given to the body of knowledge used to support nursing practice and nursing models are constructed from these theories and ideas.

Nursing models are used to help the nursing team assess, plan and implement patient care by providing a framework within which to work; they can also help the nursing team achieve uniformity and seamless continuity of care.

Nursing models are integral to the practice of nursing, providing structures that guide nurses in delivering high-quality, person-centred care. These models are theoretical frameworks that define the principles, goals and responsibilities of nursing care, emphasising holistic and individualised approaches to patient care. Nursing models have been around for a long time and found favour in the 1980s as a way of structuring care and managing nurse education; while you may not recognise that you are using a nursing model, in today's healthcare system many of our systems and processes are based on the nursing models. Understanding how a model can support nursing practice, and being able to identify the one that is most appropriate for your patients and setting will support you to structure and prioritise care.

One of the most important things when looking at developing a plan of care is to be able to justify why something is considered a priority; as a registered professional, you will need to justify the decisions you make and the care you deliver. Just as a physical model (e.g. a model of a heart) represents reality, nursing models provide a framework to understand the patient's reality. This means that nursing associates will be able to understand the reality of the patient, what their life is like, what is normal for them, how it has changed through illness or injury, what they may need support with in either the short or long term; it then allows the NA to act upon it with predictable outcomes.

Both person-centred care and nursing models agree with the following concepts of care.

- Caring is based on continuous healing relationships.
- Patients are the source and centre of care.
- Care is customised and reflects the values and needs of patients.
- Families are an integral part of the care team.
- All team members are caregivers.

- Caring is provided in an environment of comfort and support.
- Transparency is the number one rule in patient care.
- Safety is a visible care priority.
- Caregivers focus on the best interest and goals of the patient.

The multiplicity of nursing models reflects the different values and beliefs held by different communities and the individuals within them; the wider society; their health and wellbeing or indeed ill health; and the goals of planned care and support implemented. This is undertaken while also considering the roles and functions of the nursing team involved in delivering that care.

Models also represent the different needs experienced by those receiving care in the four fields of nursing and the theories that underpin them.

Popular Nursing Models

Orem (1980)

Orem states that each person is responsible for their own self-care in relation to their health; she suggests that individuals are responsible for those who are dependent on others such as children, the elderly and the sick. Orem recognises that everyone has the right to have choices regarding their health. Orem's model of self-care identifies three distinct areas of care.

Self-care requisites are what the individual can do for themselves. This part of the model is further broken down into three sections:

- 'universal self-care requisites' which focuses on maintaining the human body and its functions, including things like intake of air (breathing), intake of food and water etc. – the basic needs to keep themselves alive
- 'developmental self-care requisites', which are new requisites (needs) that have come from a condition or event such as an accident
- 'health deviation requisites' which concentrates on managing the effects of an illness, condition or disease that requires medical intervention, and also discusses how the patient sees themselves now that they have a new diagnosis.

Self-care deficits are what the individual needs support with to achieve the requisites and *nursing systems* are what needs to be put in place through nursing care delivery to ensure the individual achieves their needs.

Peplau's Theory of Nursing (1991)

Peplau's theory was first created in 1952 and was the first nursing theory to be written without a doctor as a co-author. It focuses on the interpersonal relationship between the nurse and patient and gained popularity in the field of mental health in the late 1960s. In the model, the nurse has a variety of roles: 'stranger', 'teacher', 'resource role', 'counsellor', 'surrogate' and 'leader'. Peplau identified four main phases within the interpersonal relationship: 'orientation', 'identification', 'exploitation' and 'resolution'. This model represents the journey a patient experiences and the role of the nurse in supporting that journey.

Roper, Logan and Tierney (2000)

The Roper-Logan-Tierney (RLT) model of nursing is based on the activities of living and evolved from original work by Virginia Henderson. The RLT model is widely recognised as being revolutionary in developing nursing from a bio-medical model to one which considers the patient holistically with individual needs. The model is designed to be used alongside the nursing process (see Chapter 2) and promotes a holistic approach by enabling the nursing team to identify individual needs through the exploration of 12 activities of daily living (ADLs) (maintaining a safe environment, communicating, breathing, eating and drinking, eliminating, personal cleansing and dressing, controlling body temperature, mobilising, working and playing, expressing sexuality, sleeping, dying) and what factors are affecting the person's ability to independently manage needs associated with each of these factors. Specifically, the model explores the impact of biological, psychological, sociocultural, environmental and politico-economic factors in conjunction with an individual's position on their lifespan and their independence or dependence in these activities (Holland and Jenkins 2019).

Recovery Star

The recovery star model (MacKeith and Burns 2010) is predominantly used as a tool to support service users to live well with their mental ill health, when symptoms are present and when they are not (Scottish Recovery Network 2006; Onifade 2011). Service users can use the recovery star to look at recovery as a journey with many stages; as recovery is not a straight line from end to end, service users can be supported to recognise that the journey requires change, and may require them to move back and forth within that journey. It enables them to see that their journey will be different from that of other service users (MacKeith and Burns 2010).

There are two elements to the model: the ten-point star visual diagram which maps ten areas significant to recovery (see below); and the ladder of change, which recognises five key areas that a service user will travel back and forth through as required (see below) (Onifade 2011). The ladder is present in each of the ten points, and differs in structure for each of the points but follows the same five themes.

Ten Points on the Star

- Managing mental health
- Self-care
- Living skills
- Social networks
- Work
- Relationships
- Addictive behaviours
- Responsibility
- Identity and self-esteem
- Trust and hope

Five Key Themes of the Ladder
■ Stuck ■ Accepting help ■ Believing ■ Learning ■ Self-reliant

The key feature of the model is that it is individual to each service user, and allows them to identify and focus on what matters to them most, thus supporting the ethos of person-centred care.

Other models not discussed here include:

- Henderson
- Roy's adaptation model
- Neumann.

As an NA, you should have some level of understanding of the models available to support the development of appropriate care plans, as the choice of model should be led by the needs and goals of the patient – not your preferred model or the one you understand best. You can't fit all patients into your preferred model – this in itself would work against the aims of person-centred care.

The Nursing Process

The nursing process is a foundational framework used worldwide. It involves a systematic, five-step process: assessment, diagnosis, planning, implementation and evaluation. This framework supports person-centred care by ensuring that each patient's unique health status and needs are thoroughly assessed and addressed. During the assessment phase, NAs will gather comprehensive data about the patient, including medical history, lifestyle and preferences, which are crucial for person-centred care. You will discuss all information gathered with the RN, who will make a formal assessment of the needs of the patient and make nursing diagnoses. This information will also inform the planning phase which involves the setting of individualised goals and the creation of a tailored care plan by the RN, ensuring that interventions to be delivered by the NA are specific to the patient's circumstances and wishes.

Effective communication and shared decision making are crucial. NAs can engage patients in discussions about their care options, listen to their concerns and preferences, and involve them in setting care goals. This collaborative approach ensures that care plans are aligned with what is important to the patient.

You will be involved in building trusting relationships with patients, demonstrating empathy and providing emotional support. This approach helps patients feel valued and understood, which is essential for person-centred care.

Implementing nursing models to support person-centred care is not without challenges. You may face barriers such as time constraints, high patient workload and limited resources. Additionally, cultural differences and language barriers can complicate communication and understanding between nurses and patients.

Despite the challenges, commitment to person-centred care remains a fundamental principle of nursing, reflecting the profession's dedication to recognising and respecting the needs and preferences of each patient.

Patient and Family-centred Care

Historically, family-centred care (FCC) had its roots firmly within children's healthcare services but with no clear definition as such and is now increasingly recognised in, and adapted to other fields of practice (Mikkelson and Frederiksen 2011).

There are three main principles of FCC.

- That a child is only admitted to hospital if the care they require cannot be provided at home – mainly by the family.
- That FCC is clearly explained and understood by the family and nurses/carers, so that they can discuss and negotiate their roles.
- That FCC is implemented in such a way as to consider all elements of family life.

An effective partnership exists when nurses, NAs, carers and healthcare providers recognise that parents are often the experts in caring for their children, and particularly in the case of children with long-term and complex health conditions.

There are barriers to the effective provision of FCC. There may be other children to look after and therefore parents will need to balance care needs for all. Parents may need to take time off work to bring children for appointments or admissions and this may mean losing pay and increased stress. Parents may have their own health concerns or needs, affecting their ability to understand information given or to be present or participate in their child's care. Healthcare may need to be accessed from a significant distance, particularly when specialist services is provided in regional or national centres, and this may mean the child is a long way from home, impacting on finances, stress and the ability to function as a family unit.

Studies have shown that health professionals do not always recognise that parents are the expert in their child's health and care needs, preferring to assume that parents do not have the specialist training and expertise to fully understand or make decisions in the best interests of the child, and that these decisions should be left to the health professionals. Others have the opinion that while parents should be informed of decisions made regarding their child's health, the final decision should rest with the professional.

Patient and family-centred care (PFCC) recognises the importance of the patient's family members and the role they play in planning for discharge as well as planning care to meet needs at home. The principles of PFCC include listening to families, facilitating choice, sharing information and building confidence to participate in healthcare decision making. By implementing PFCC, clinicians benefit by gathering more information, improving follow-through, making efficient use of professional time and decreased healthcare utilisation (Point of Care Foundation 2024).

As an NA, your role is pivotal in ensuring that the needs of the family are met. Until you understand the needs and goals of a family, it is impossible to ensure that care is family centred. Being placed 'at the bedside' allows the NA to build an effective working relationship with the family as well as the patient; this creates trust and allows the patient and their family to be open and honest about their fears, hopes, potential lack of understanding and previous experiences, in order to develop realistic and achievable care plans.

There are several barriers to PFCC that you may come across as an NA. One that parents and carers find difficult to understand, in the UK, is that they do not have the automatic right to have access to their child's medical notes; that they will have to apply for access and that this may take several months to be agreed. This may be described as counterproductive to a relationship that requires trust and mutual respect, as those requesting access may feel that they are being denied this as the caregivers have something to hide. Other barriers include, but are not limited to, a breakdown in communication or a recognised communication barrier such as language, hearing loss or inability to speak; fear; addressing safeguarding concerns, and the trauma this may cause when confronting concerns which may lead to a breakdown in family dynamics – particularly when different members of the family do not agree on the same approach. These are only a few barriers – you may come across many more throughout your career and you may need to adapt your interpersonal skills to manage them.

The implementation of FCC has numerous benefits for patients, families and healthcare providers.

- *Improved outcomes*: patients often experience better health outcomes, including shorter hospital stays, reduced readmissions and enhanced recovery.
- *Enhanced satisfaction*: patients report higher satisfaction with their care when their families are involved and their preferences are respected.
- *Increased compliance*: patients are more likely to adhere to treatment plans when their families are engaged and supportive.
- *Empowerment*: families feel more empowered and confident in their ability to care for their loved ones.
- *Reduced anxiety*: knowing they are a vital part of the team can reduce stress and anxiety for family members.
- *Better understanding*: families gain a better understanding of the patient's condition and treatment which can improve at-home care.
- *Improved relationships*: providers develop stronger, more trusting relationships with patients and families.
- *Enhanced communication*: open lines of communication lead to fewer misunderstandings and better overall care.
- *Professional satisfaction*: providers often experience greater job satisfaction when they work collaboratively with families.

Person-centred Care at End of Life

Delivering end-of-life care in a person-centred way is a cornerstone of nursing practice. This approach ensures that the needs, preferences and values of the patient and their families are respected and prioritised. Person-centred care and end-of-life care both involve a holistic understanding of the patient, effective communication, empathy and the provision of compassionate support. By focusing on pain management, emotional support, cultural sensitivity and ethical considerations, you can provide high-quality care that respects the individual needs and preferences of patients and their families. Respecting patient autonomy and ensuring informed consent are essential. Patients should be empowered to make decisions about their care, and their choices should be respected, even if they differ from the preferences of their family or healthcare team.

Nursing associates should practise active listening, which involves giving full attention to the patient, acknowledging their feelings and responding appropriately. This can help patients feel heard and valued, which is particularly important during the emotional and often stressful end-of-life phase. When discussing prognosis and care options, it is important that you communicate clearly and compassionately. You should avoid medical jargon and provide information in a way that is understandable to the patient and their family. This helps them to make informed decisions about care preferences.

Facilitating discussions about advance care planning is another key aspect. This involves talking about the patient's wishes regarding treatment options, resuscitation preferences and other end-of-life care decisions. By discussing these matters early, nurses can ensure that the patient's preferences are known and respected when they might no longer be able to communicate them.

Effective pain and symptom management is essential in person-centred end-of-life care. Ensuring that the patient is as comfortable as possible can significantly improve the quality of life in their final days. Regularly evaluating your patient's pain and symptoms is crucial. You should use appropriate pain assessment tools and scales to understand the intensity and nature of the pain as this will guide the appropriate interventions.

Being involved in the development of individualised pain management plans that are tailored to the patient's specific needs and preferences is essential. Working in a multidisciplinary team, including doctors, palliative care specialists and pain management experts, can help create a comprehensive pain management strategy. Being the NA at the bedside, you have optimum opportunity to fully understand your patient and how they want their pain managed. This may include using pharmacological interventions, such as opioids and non-opioid pain medications, as well as non-pharmacological methods like heat or ice packs, massage, relaxation techniques and acupuncture. NAs can facilitate access to counselling services and support groups. These resources can help patients and families cope with the emotional challenges of the end-of-life phase. Nurses can also refer patients to mental health professionals when necessary.

Addressing spiritual needs is also important. For many patients, spirituality or religious beliefs play a significant role in their end-of-life experience. Nurses should respect and support these beliefs, whether by facilitating visits from spiritual leaders, providing resources or simply offering a listening ear.

Person-centred end-of-life care involves addressing not only the physical needs of the patient but also their emotional, social and spiritual needs. This holistic approach ensures comprehensive care that respects the individuality of the patient. As an NA, you should work with the RN in developing personalised care plans that reflect the unique needs and preferences of the patient. These plans should consider the patient's medical condition, personal values and goals of care. They should cover the use of holistic therapies, such as music therapy, art therapy and pet therapy, where available, as they can enhance the quality of life for end-of-life patients. If you are not able to care for your patient in their own home, then creating a comfortable and soothing environment is important. Ensuring that the patient's room is peaceful, with personal items and photos, can create a more home-like and comforting atmosphere.

Providing support and education to family members is essential. NAs can offer guidance on how to care for the patient, manage symptoms and navigate the emotional challenges of the end-of-life phase. This support can help families feel more confident and involved in the care process. Families play a critical role in supporting the patient and making care decisions. Regular family meetings can help keep the family informed about the patient's condition and care plan. These meetings provide an opportunity for family members to ask questions, express concerns and participate in decision making.

Offering bereavement support to families after the patient's death is also important. This can include counselling services, support groups and resources to help families cope with their loss. Involving the family in the care process is a key aspect of person-centred end-of-life care

Supporting Person-centred Care with Cultural Competence

Cultural competence in nursing is the ability of healthcare providers to recognise and respect the cultural backgrounds, values, beliefs and practices of their patients. This competence is essential in delivering high-quality healthcare in diverse societies. Health inequalities among different cultural groups are a significant concern in healthcare and cultural competence in nursing helps address these disparities by ensuring that all patients receive equitable care. In nursing, cultural competence involves understanding the cultural differences that affect health behaviours and medical practices, improving patient outcomes and satisfaction.

The importance of cultural competence in nursing cannot be overstated. As our communities become increasingly multicultural, NAs are likely to encounter patients from various cultural backgrounds. Cultural competence helps NAs provide care that is person centred and respects each patient's unique cultural needs, resulting in improved patient trust, communication and overall care quality. This is particularly crucial in preventing misunderstandings.

Effective communication is the cornerstone of quality healthcare, allowing NAs to communicate effectively with patients from different cultural backgrounds; by understanding and respecting cultural differences, NAs can bridge communication gaps, ensuring that patients understand their diagnoses, treatment options and care plans. Patients who feel understood and respected by their healthcare providers are more likely to be satisfied with their care.

Cultural competence helps NAs build trust and rapport with patients, making them feel valued and respected. This positive relationship fosters an environment where patients are more willing to share vital information about their health, leading to more accurate diagnoses and effective person-centred care plans.

Cultural competence in nursing comprises five key components: cultural awareness, cultural knowledge, cultural skill, cultural encounters and cultural desire (Stubbe 2020).

Cultural Awareness

Cultural awareness involves recognising the cultural differences and similarities that exist among patients. As an NA, you must be aware of your own cultural biases and prejudices to provide unbiased care. This self-awareness will help you to avoid imposing your own cultural values on patients and allows you to respect the cultural values of others.

Cultural Knowledge

Cultural knowledge entails understanding the cultural practices, beliefs and values of different patient populations. This knowledge can be gained through education, training and direct interaction with diverse cultural groups. As an NA, you will need cultural knowledge to ensure you are better equipped to understand the health-related behaviours and needs of your patients.

Cultural Skill

Cultural skill is the ability to conduct cultural assessments and gather relevant cultural information about patients. This skill enables you to tailor your care to meet the specific cultural needs of your patients. For example, understanding a patient's dietary restrictions based on their cultural or religious practices can help you to provide appropriate nutritional advice and care.

Cultural Encounters

Cultural encounters refer to the direct interactions between NAs and patients from diverse cultural backgrounds. These encounters provide opportunities for you to apply your cultural knowledge and skills in real-world settings. Through these interactions, you can develop greater cultural competence and learn to navigate the complexities of cross-cultural healthcare.

Cultural Desire

Cultural desire is the genuine motivation to become culturally competent. It involves a willingness to learn about different cultures and to engage with patients from diverse backgrounds with empathy and respect. Cultural desire drives you to continually improve your cultural competence and provide the best possible care to all patients.

Despite its importance, achieving cultural competence in nursing presents challenges. These challenges can hinder the delivery of culturally competent, person-centred care and in turn impact patient outcomes. Language barriers are one of the most significant challenges in providing culturally competent care. Patients with limited proficiency in the English language may struggle to communicate their symptoms, understand medical instructions and express their concerns. As an NA, you must find effective ways to overcome these barriers, such as using professional interpreters or translation services.

Stereotyping and prejudices can negatively affect the nurse–patient relationship. You must be vigilant in recognising and addressing your biases to providing equitable care. This involves ongoing self-reflection and education to challenge and change prejudiced attitudes. The fast-paced nature of healthcare can make it difficult for you to spend the necessary time understanding and addressing the cultural needs of your patients. Time constraints can lead to a more task-oriented approach to care, which may overlook the cultural dimensions of person-centred care. Despite the challenges in achieving cultural competence, strategies such as education and training, use of interpreters, development of cultural assessment tools, encouraging cultural encounters and promoting cultural desire can help you to provide person-centred, culturally competent care.

Chapter Summary

Person-centred care is the goal, and is achievable, but it requires effort and that begins with an understanding of what being person centred really means, how we deliver it and how we evaluate its effectiveness. There needs to be an understanding of the patient's or service user's needs; an agreement on the goals; there needs to be effort in provision of choice and treatment options; care plans need to be developed with the wider nursing and multidisciplinary teams, that take into account those preferences and choices; there needs to be ongoing communication with the patient or service user with evaluation of how effective plans are, and the progression made; and we should be seen to be responsive to feedback given.

References

Department of Health and Social Care (2021). Guidance – NHS Constitution for England. www.gov.uk/government/publications/the–nhs–constitution–for–england

Francis, R. (2013). *Inquiry Report into Mid Staffordshire NHS Foundation Trust*. London: Stationery Office.

Hardy, S. (2015). Perspectives: is health and social care person centred? Hello, my name is not enough. *Journal of Research in Nursing* 20 (6): 517–522.

Harris, M. (2021). *Understanding Person-Centred Care for Nursing Associates*. Thousand Oaks: Sage.

Health Foundation (2016). *Person-Centred Care Made Simple: What Everyone Should Know about Person-Centred Care*. London: Health Foundation.

Holland, K. and Jenkins, J. (2019). *Applying the Roper-Logan-Tierney Model in Practice.*, 3e. London: Elsevier.

Kirkup, B. (2015). *The Report of the Morecambe Bay Investigation*. London: Stationery Office.

MacKeith, J. and Burns, S. (2010). The Recovery Star: User Guide. 2e. https://mnpmind. org.uk/wp-content/uploads/2021/09/Recovery-STAR--Guide.pdf

McCormack, B. and McCance, T. (ed.) (2016). *Person-Centred Practice in Nursing and Health Care: Theory and Practice*, 2e. Chichester: John Wiley & Sons.

Mikkelsen, G. and Frederiksen, K. (2011). Family-centred care of children in hospital – a concept analysis. *Journal of Advanced Nursing* 65 (5): 1152–1162.

NHS (2019). NHS Long Term Plan. www.longtermplan.nhs.uk

NHS England (2014). NHS Five Year Forward View. www.england.nhs.uk/wp-content/uploads/2014/10/5yfv-web.pdf

Nursing and Midwifery Council (2018). *Standards of Proficiency for Nursing Associates*. London: NMC.

Onifade, Y. (2011). The mental health recovery star. *Mental Health and Social Inclusion* 15 (2): 78–87.

Orem, D.E. (1980). *Nursing : Concepts of Practice*. New York: Mcgraw Hill.

Peate, I. (2019). *Learning to Care: The Nursing Associate*. London: Elsevier.

Peplau, H. (1991). *Interpersonal Relations in Nursing: A Conceptual Frame of Reference for Psychodynamic Nursing*. New York: Springer.

Point of Care Foundation (2024). What is PFCC and why is it needed? www.pointof carefoundation.org.uk/resource/patient-family-centred-care-toolkit/introduction/what-is-pfcc-and-why-is-it-needed/

Roper, N., Logan, W., and Tierney, A. (2000). *The Roper-Logan-Tierney Model of Nursing: Based on Activities of Daily Living*. London: Churchill Livingstone.

Scottish Recovery Network (2006) Journeys of Recovery: Stories of Hope and Recovery from Long-term Mental Health. www.scottishrecovery.net

Smith, J.B. and Willis, E. (2020). Interpreting posthumanism with nurse work. *Journal of Posthuman Studies* 4 (1): 59–75.

Stubbe, D.E. (2020). Practicing cultural competence and cultural humility in the care of diverse patients. *Focus* 18 (1): 49–51.

Further Reading

Brooker, D. and Latham, I. (2016). *Person-Centred Dementia Care: Making Services Better with the VIPS Framework*, 2e. London: Jessica Kingsley.

Campinha-Bacote, J. (2003). Cultural desire: the key to unlocking cultural competence. *Journal of Nursing Education* 42 (6): 239–240.

Fox, D. and Wilson, D. (1999). Parents' experiences of general hospital admissions for adults with learning disabilities. *Journal of Clinical Nursing* 8: 610–614.

Grant, A. and Goodman, B. (2019). *Communication and Interpersonal Skills in Nursing*, 4e. London: Sage/Learning Matters.

Health Foundation (2024). Patient and Family Centred Care www.health.org.uk/funding-and-partnerships/programmes/patient-and-family-centred-care

Howatson-Jones, L., Standing, M., and Roberts, S. (2015). *Patient Assessment and Care Planning in Nursing*, 2e. London: Sage.

Kitwood, T. (1997). *Dementia Reconsidered: The Person Comes First*. Buckingham.: Open University Press.

Kokorelias, K., Gignac, M., Naglie, G., and Cameron, J. (2019). Towards a universal model of family centred care: a scoping review. *BMC Health Services Research* 19: 564.

Kuo, D.Z., Houtrow, A.J., Arango, P. et al. (2012). Family-centered care: current applications and future directions in pediatric health care. *Maternal and Child Health Journal* 16 (2): 297–305.

Lee, K., Lee, J., and Kim, B. (2022). Person-centered care in persons living with dementia: a systematic review and meta-analysis. *Gerontologist* 62 (4): e253–e264.

Li, J. and Porock, D. (2014). Resident outcomes of person-centered care in long-term care: a narrative review of interventional research. *International Journal of Nursing Studies* 51 (10): 1395–1415.

McCormack, B., Dewing, J., and McCance, T. (2011). Developing person-centred care: addressing contextual challenges through practice development. *Online Journal of Issues in Nursing* 16 (2): 3.

Nicol, J. and Nyatanga, B. (2017). *Palliative and End of Life Care in Nursing*. London: Learning Matters.

Nursing and Midwifery Council (NMC) (2018). *The Code. Standards of Practice and Behaviour for Nurses Midwives and Nursing Associates*. London: Nursing and Midwifery Council.

Nursing and Midwifery Council (NMC) (2020). We regulate nursing associates. www.nmc.org.uk/about-us/our-role/who-we-regulate/nursing-associates/

Orem, D. (2001). *Nursing: Concepts of Practice*. Philadelphia: Lippincott Williams and Wilkins.

Pepper, A. and Harrison Dening, K. (2023). Person-centred communication with people with dementia. *Nursing Older People* 35 (2).

Purssell, E. and Sagoo, R. (2023). Children's care: family centred but child focused. *British Journal of Nursing* 32 (10): 466–470.

Roberts, J., Fenton, G., and Barnard, M. (2015). Developing effective therapeutic relationships with children, young people and their families. *Nursing Children and Young People* 27 (4): 30–35.

Roper, N. (1976). *Clinical Experience in Nurse Education*. London: Churchill Livingstone.

Wheeler, N. and Gardner, R. (2016). A wellbeing tool to help plan care for older people. *Nursing Times* 112 (39): 21–24.

5 Effective Communication for the Nursing Associate

Michelle Richardson

University Hospitals of Leicester NHS Trust, Leicester, UK

Introduction

The registered nursing associate (NA) role is essential in supporting health individuality, gaining trust and ensuring that the patient voice is recognised as integral to care. Interpersonal relationships are fundamental to competent delivery of healthcare (Cox 2018). This chapter will focus on developing these skills post registration and will consider the principles taught during the programme in relation to the NMC Standards (NMC 2018) and how these can be developed. Attention will be paid to the NA role in activities such as breaking bad news, developing a multidisciplinary approach to managing language barriers and developing effective relationships.

Aims of This Chapter

- To identify and take a compassionate response towards individual communication styles.
- To recognise the factors that influence an individual's ability to communicate.
- To identify our own communication skills, and areas where we need to develop our confidence in communication.

Related to NMC Standards

Demonstrate an understanding of the communication and interpersonal skills of a nursing associate as defined in Annexe A of the NMC Standards.

Explain the importance of clear and effective communication with regard to person-centred care, duty of care, candour, equality and diversity (1.9).

Describe a range of techniques and strategies and the principles underpinning them that promote clear and effective communication (1.10).

Demonstrate the ability to act as an ambassador for the nursing associate profession and promote public confidence in health and care services (1.16).

The Importance of 'Good' Communication

Communication forms a connection between two people or a group of people, it establishes goals, barriers and commonalities and it humanises those involved. Communication ensures that person-centred care is being acknowledged; person-centred care would not be possible without communication. Good communication ensures that the person feels listened to and is part of their care journey. Patient satisfaction increases when patients are not just communicated to but listened to, which in turn improves co-operation with treatment plans. Maguire and Pitceathly (2002) wrote that all those involved benefit when communication is undertaken well in healthcare. Communication will also be present within the professional relationship between colleagues, with good communication in this context ensuring consistent care with all involved providing their expertise.

As a registrant, you may find yourself as the most experienced person within your clinical area supporting individuals with mental health problems, young people or those in pain or at the end of life. There may be an expectation for you to step forward and take a lead in these scenarios, and it will be your responsibility to not only communicate but support your colleagues in developing their communication skills.

Evidence-based communication is closely interwoven with theory and personal development. It is not a skill that you can learn from a textbook or a PowerPoint, it is about learning to observe, listen and being honest about yourself. Communication comes from interaction after interaction, embracing meeting with others, listening to their stories and understanding who they are and the experiences that shape them. It is about connection.

The role of the NA is also to recognise the diversity of our patients and service users and how that diversity will impact on how someone communicates and their needs for good communication. For the remainder of this chapter, patients and service users will be identified as 'service users'.

The life stage of a person will change the way they communicate, due not just to age but also their life experiences, emotional literacy and changing physical health. Although this chapter is broken into distinct subheadings, this does not mean that someone will present exclusively with one barrier, and your role as an NA is to recognise the variability of this.

Underpinning Theories

The theoretical basis of communication provides the foundations to good communication. Reading and understanding the underpinning theories will aid you to observe and reflect on why an interaction went well, or not, and suggests how you could approach this interaction in a different way. In terms of evidence basis, the term 'theoretical consensus' is used, which justifies the lack of position on the hierarchy of evidence (see Chapter 8 for more detail). Theoretical consensus refers to the collaborative involvement of peers, whereby an expert within a field presents their theory based on a collection of data, and fellow experts within that or similar fields present a conclusion to agree or disagree with the proposed theory. As discussed within Chapter 3, nursing is an art as well as a science and with this in mind, observing human behaviour and understanding this would be an art.

Specific theories that identify communicative behaviours, such as those of Shannon and Weaver (1949) and Mehrabian (1971), present grounded theories for how humans communicate and the behaviours they exhibit. However, with theoretical consensus comes the opportunity to critique and challenge ideas. Over the following decades, criticism has been raised as to how the blanket approaches of these theories often do not consider the distinct nuances that each person presents. For example, predecessors of Shannon and Weaver (Berlo 1960; Stead 1972) presented humanistic elements to their adaptation of the model, while Hall (1966) introduced the role proximity has on interaction and emotional investment. These authors sought to demonstrate that the needs within the communication episode are dictated by the situation, such as being work related, but also the focus and engagement in the conversation topic will be influenced by the person's needs (i.e. if the conversation does not meet a need, or that need is already achieved, the receiver will not engage).

Following on from understanding communication, we then need to think about how we use this knowledge to build the therapeutic relationship. Peplau (1991) presented a model that looked beyond the specific behaviours of communication, and proposed that we acknowledge the situation that person is in, where you take your time with a relationship, not rushing to be the dominant 'all-knowing' professional but rather getting to know the other person, learning who they are, where they have been and where they want to go (see Chapter 4 for further information on Peplau). Only when you know each other in the therapeutic sense should you then explore what you can do for that person.

Reflective Activity: What the Word "Communication" Means to You

Consider the following questions in relation to your experiences with patients, carers and service users.

- What is communication?
- Why do we need effective communication?
- What qualities do you have to facilitate effective communication?

Understanding Ourselves and How We Develop Our Own Communication

Before trying to understand why your service user communicates in a particular way, it is necessary to understand your own communication style. Assessment and diagnosis of another person's behaviour need to come from a place of self-awareness. Self-awareness is key in recognising how your presence impacts others around you; are you aloof so that people will not open up emotionally but will come to you to resolve situations efficiently, or are you gentle so people feel they can share their challenges but would not turn to you for support in aggressive conflict?

To begin, we will explore where personality and communication styles come from and apply that to yourself. We will use the analogy of a house to represent our own personality.

The House Analogy

Foundations

The foundations are the elements that will influence your personality before you are born. This may be due to your parents' actions during gestation, such as diet, substance use (legal, illegal or prescribed) and trauma the parent experiences such as accident, injury or abuse; these present significant risks to fetal development or poor mental health in later life. You may also be impacted by intergenerational trauma (Danieli 1998), where trauma experienced by your grandparents or parents will impact on your mental health, through fear, anxiety and confidence. There are also the positive elements, such as your parents' culture, where open and constructive communication is celebrated, where gender and personal identity barriers are not present. Genetics will also affect your foundations. There is evidence of genetic links with certain mental health conditions, but in turn there will be genetic protection from other conditions.

The Airbricks

The airbricks represent the birthing experience. If a child is going to be diagnosed with a learning disability, there must be evidence that it was present pre-birth or occurred during the birthing process. Children born preterm are at increased risk of being diagnosed with learning and attention differences, which will impact on their confidence and communication skills. Other birth traumas that happen to the baby, such as significant injury, can affect confidence and relationship development. The potential for the parent to experience post-traumatic stress disorder (PTSD) from the birthing experience has been observed and this in turn has links to the parents' ability to bond with their baby. There is increasing awareness of the trauma experienced by the birthing partner, which may also impact on bonding with that parent.

The Walls, Windows and Door

This is the childhood experience, which could include adverse childhood events (ACEs), bullying, positive parenting, emotional awareness, significant social events such as war, poverty and social exclusion. This also includes attachment, such as Bowlby's Theory of Attachment (1958), where the first six months of life are crucial in forming bonds which affect later life.

Educational experience and attainment will also inform confidence and awareness in later life.

The Roof

This is the final part of the house and represents adulthood. Again, there are many theories of when your identity fully forms, from 26 years old to 80 years. Regardless, this will be influenced by your educational attainment, relationships (familial, friendship and partnerships), vocational route and experience. Your working experience, the culture you work in and the community of practice you learn from will role model communication and engagement with a range of different people in varied circumstances. Your ability to travel and experience other cultures as an adult will also be influential.

Once you have reflected on your own life experiences, you may find you can pinpoint events in your life – a specific encounter with a colleague, a culturally enlightening event or a lifelong situation – that have had significant influences on how you communicate.

Now is the time to pay attention to yourself; think about your own behaviours, responses and mannerisms, which you demonstrate when you communicate. Are you a confident, relaxed communicator or anxious and avoid potential conflict? How does your communication or response influence how others communicate with you? The Johari Window (see below) is an activity to complete around self-awareness and think about how you might apply this to a person you are struggling to communicate with.

Reflective Activity: Johari Window

The Johari Window is an exercise in understanding yourself. Write the window out yourself and fill out the panes. Think about the feedback you have received from others and the opinions you hold on yourself to build this window. A Johari Window is personal but it is a tool for identifying the parts of you that you are comfortable to share and the parts that remain private.

	Known to self	Unknown to self
Known to others	**Open Self:** Information about you that both you and others know	**Blind Self:** Information about you that you do not know but others do know
Unknown to others	**Hidden Self:** Information about you that you know but others do not	**Unknown Self:** Information about you that neither you nor others know

Now that you have reviewed yourself and what makes you who you are, how do we acknowledge this and reflect on our own communication skills? And how do we identify the impact this has on others around us? Woodbridge and Fulford (2004) stated that we all carry our own values and experiences, and we need to recognise where ours will match or contradict those of our patients, and how we can ensure that ours do not influence our service users negatively. We all have personal values which are embedded in our personalities, but which of these are appropriate to display in work in order to humanise ourselves, and which should we keep private?

The Johari Window demonstrates that parts of our self will be displayed to others and others will remain private. The activity below is an exercise in identifying which parts you are happy to open and exposed, which you keep private, and what other people have fed back to you. Once you have completed the activity, take some time to reflect on what you have written – are you satisfied with this or would you prefer to come across a different way, and has the feedback you have received from others come from a place of support or negativity? Reflection may lead to change, but it can also lead to reassurance that you are bringing out your most authentic self.

You will not be the only professional communicating within your practice area, and observing others' communication styles is helpful in developing our own. The Hidden Curriculum (Giroux and Penna 1983; Cruess et al. 2016) says that we learn to communicate through our ongoing life experiences and as we develop our identity (both personal and professional), we develop our ability to communicate with others. This will be based on the people we have communicated with (colleagues, friends, the public). Specifically within education, Giroux and Penna (1983) explored how communication skills are learnt from your surroundings (classroom or workplace) and not explicitly through textbooks and the teaching on the board. This concept means that you will have observed and experienced others' interactions and have reflected (actively and passively) on these to shape your own communication styles. For example, if we are continuously exposed to conflict-based communication in the workplace, this is what we will learn as the norm, as with passive and avoidant communication. However, if we are exposed to a variety of communication styles at work, we will reflect and identify which approaches work best in different situations and will emulate that behaviour.

> **Reflective Activity: Observing Practice**
>
> An activity to take back into practice: observing others' behaviours, how they use body language and conversational prompts to encourage dialogue.

Developing an Effective Therapeutic Relationship

Careful cultivation of a variety of communication skills and methods is necessary in building a trusting collaborative relationship between the professional and the client. The nurse–patient relationship stems from preconceived ideas of roles and responsibilities with expectations already laid out; however, these are generic towards a set profession and a set client group. The therapeutic relationship follows on from this stage, and is built on mutual growth and learning between one professional and one client.

Peplau's theory of interpersonal relations, the development of the therapeutic relationship, says that through communication there are stages that must be followed to develop the relationship – however, this assumes that there is significant time to do so. In situations where time is limited, the nurse–patient relationship must be followed. When time is short, particularly in assessment, emergency and admission areas, trust and co-operation must be built quickly and efficiently.

The professional needs to take steps to establish what the client wants to achieve and what is achievable in a short space of time. You may not have time to fully consider the person's developmental journey, and instead focus on key elements to communication, such as age, culture and disability. These elements will all influence the service user's predisposed attitude towards working with professionals. They may hold a hierarchical attitude towards professionals, identifying the NA as less knowledgeable or of less significance than a doctor or sister/charge nurse. Alternatively, they may have prior positive experience of with working with a NA which leads them to identify you as the most trusted advocate for their care. Stewart et al. (2015) identified that patients, service users or clients have a preconceived perception of the staff they come across, so it is our responsibility to acknowledge this, through considering their past experiences, then introducing them to a new style of communication and relationship for this new professional.

> ■ **Key learning point:** do not make assumptions about someone's communication barriers or needs – use your full assessment skills (ask the person, ask the carer, read the notes and document) to fully establish the impact a barrier has on their communication and what adjustments you need to be making.

Influential factors such as those above, and ones we will explore in the rest of the chapter, draw together the argument for holism. Holism is the method of considering the person as a whole, with their biological, psychological and social needs and wants influencing their care. This again draws on the analogy of the house presented earlier in the chapter. When approaching someone to initiate your care process, they will not be simply communicating to you in a particular style, they will be communicating with past life experience, formed from comfort, support, frustration and hostility. Acknowledging that individual's background, demonstrating unconditional positive regard and communicating yourself with empathy, honesty and self-awareness will demonstrate to them that you are safe to communicate with.

Another factor to consider in developing the therapeutic relationship is understanding how service users express their emotions, and how confident they are in communicating this. Emotional intelligence is described as the ability to perceive, understand, manage and use emotions in self and others (Cox 2018). How service users or carers express their emotions will in turn affect how they communicate their needs to you. The framework of Salovey and Mayer (1990) demonstrates the factors that influence someone's ability to express self-awareness and social awareness.

> **Emotional Intelligence**
>
> ■ *Perceived emotions*: understanding what an emotion is and what it means.
> ■ *Managing emotions*: being able to express emotions without causing increased distress to self.
> ■ *Facilitating thought using emotions*: being able to verbalise what the emotion means and express this clearly to others.
> ■ *Understanding emotions*: ability to recognise what has triggered an emotion and not another.

Using Communication to Engage and Develop Care

Once a relationship is established, whether that is the nurse–patient relationship or the more in-depth therapeutic relationship, the natural progression is to establish what the mutual goals of the relationship will be and the roles which you will both play in this.

Maguire and Pitceathly (2002) suggest that a clinical conversation needs to elicit three main points: (i) the patient's main problems; (ii) the patient's perceptions of these; and (iii) the physical, emotional and social impact of the patient's problems on the patient and family. These three points acknowledge that communication outcomes are based on holistic, human needs, not just physical or clinical needs.

Heron's (2001) Six-stage Interventional Analysis

The way in which you communicate will be influenced by the situation you are in and the outcomes that need to be achieved. Heron (2001) says that depending on the needed outcome from the conversation, the professional will adjust the style of their delivery to match.

Heron's six-stage interventional analysis

Authoritative	Facilitative
Prescriptive – the clinician gives instructions to the patient to change. May or may not ask opinion, and opinion may or may not be relevant.	Cathartic – encouraging the client to identify and express feelings, with the aim of discharging emotions.
Informative – you provide the client with information relevant to the task you are going to carry out for their care.	Catalytic – aim to elicit self-discovery and explore own values and motivations.
Confronting – identifying behaviour, challenging the behaviour and advising change.	Supportive – instilling positive affirmations to the client to support them in identifying their self-worth.

Each of the six stages will lend itself to different scenarios, but there are scenarios in which if the wrong style is used, the consequences may be significant. Look at the example below and consider which approach would suit best, and which approach would be inappropriate and would be detrimental to health or the relationship. Use this opportunity to reflect on when you have seen similar situations occur, and which style of communication was used and what the outcomes of these were.

Example of situation	
Your client has been rude to a colleague at lunch time.	Confronting
There is a fire in the neighbouring department which requires evacuation.	Prescriptive
'You did really well at that task, you are very capable of managing this.'	Supportive
You are about to administer an IM depot to your patient.	Informative
Your client has identified that they want to make a change but need your support in thinking about how to manage this.	Catalytic
'Tell me about that event last week, how did that make you feel?'	Cathartic

Miller and Rollnick's (2012) motivational interviewing takes a coaching approach which, similar to Heron's facilitative–catalytic method, is about asking the person open questions to make them lead the direction and decision taking in their own care. A method that was initiated in addiction services, it has been used successfully to support those who have been diagnosed with a long-term condition, such as diabetes and Crohn's disease, to identify lifestyle changes that they feel are achievable. This relies on a person-centred approach to change, where the healthcare professional facilitates the changes needed and does not prescribe.

Recognised Barriers to Effective Communication

There are a broad range of communication barriers which will be influenced by the biological, psychological and social needs of the individual. We will address some of these barriers below and the skills and tools needed to support these. However, this list is in no way exhaustive, and you will find that many of the tools and approaches discussed can be applied to other communication barriers.

The ability to assess someone's communication barrier is key in meeting their needs. Towards the end of the chapter, you will be encouraged to explore the use of the nursing process (ADPIE) for each of the barriers, but as you read through each stage, reflect on your own practice and the approaches you have taken. It is also important to note that diagnosis in communication is not about diagnosing their health needs but their communication need and you as the NA are capable of completing this stage.

Communicating with Children

Communicating with children does not necessarily have to be within a children's department; it may be a GP practice or they have come in with their parents. The role of the NA is ideally suited for these unexpected interactions as the skills you bring will be creative and practised in application.

As previously discussed, communication skills develop from birth and although the average speech age is from 12 months, a child will use body language and other noises to communicate from birth. A child's communication development will be influenced by multiple factors, based on physical health, emotional development and socialisation. Thus, children will all develop their communication and confidence to communicate differently – you may have cared for a very confident, chatty four year old but that does not mean that the next four year old will communicate similarly.

Influencial Factors

There are many specific factors that will influence a child's communication. Can you identify any more that you have noted in practice?

- Age
- Prematurity at birth
- Genetic conditions
- Conditions related to physical development
- Attachment
- Neglect or abuse
- Pain
- Fear

Tools to Aid Communication

As a child develops in age, it is anticipated that they will have a wider communication set and thus be able to give you a more detailed reflection of their experience. As such, tools to aid assessment change depending on the child's communication ability. The pain assessment scales, such as Wong–Baker FACES Scale® or FLACC Scale, offer flexibility for the healthcare professional to meet the child's specific needs.

Review the Wong–Baker FACES Scale used for children aged three years and over (https://wongbakerfaces.org) and the FLACC Scale (Malviya et al. 2006) (https://media.gosh.nhs.uk/documents/Revised_FLACC_Paperwork.doc.pdf) which can provide you with greater levels of detail.

These tools can also be used collaboratively; a child may be able to identify where they feel they sit on the FACES scale but struggle to give more detail. Your ability to observe the child using the FLACC Scale will then potentially give you more detail, especially if you have engage the child in an activity.

Making use of the wider multidisciplinary team is invaluable. Play specialists will not just be to distract a child but aid communication through games and role play. A child may not be able to verbalise discomfort, but careful observation of their movement, or reluctance to move, during play can narrow down concerns. Using tools such as storytelling, puppets, drawing or books can support the child in communicating, and you sharing information back with them to their level.

You will also need to consider the parent's communication style, and how you will need to adapt to them. The presence of high expressed emotions, such as fear and anger, is increased due to the vulnerability we attach to our own child and the need to protect. Parents in this situation may not be reliable history givers due to their inability to focus on a conversation and recall accurate events. Building the therapeutic relationship is necessary to reassure the parents of the safety of their child and your compassion towards their situation – the parent will be experiencing guilt regardless of the circumstances but reassurance and support from you as the professional will develop trust and open communication channels. Parents may also present as hostile and aggressive, and although certain behaviours are not to be condoned, careful reflection on the reasons behind their behaviour is necessary.

From the age of about eight years, if there are no other influential factors, you should expect a child to verbally explain what they are experiencing and hold a conversation. However, this does not mean that they will understand what is going on, and how interventions and treatments work. Gillick Competence, the understanding that a person under the age of 16 years can consent to their own treatment without parental involvement if they have the capacity, does not have a lower age limit but it is most relevant for those 13 years and above. Judging how much you explain to a child about their health may follow from a discussion with the parents, and a staged approach to sharing.

- 'Why do you think you have come to the hospital today?'
- 'Do you know what is going to happen while you are here in hospital?'
- 'How long do you think you will be in hospital for?'

Questions such as these allow you to measure their understanding. They may have been well prepared and any procedure will not come as a surprise but if the child has not been told what to expect or has not been able to demonstrate their understanding, your preparation needs to include the potential for confusion and distress. Again, play specialist techniques can be implemented to prepare or distract the child. Utilising Social Stories (as discussed later in the chapter) can prepare the child in a way that makes them feel they are part of the process, and the use of images and written language to their literacy level means the child can utilise the resource for reassurance on their own terms.

Cultural Awareness

T.S. Eliot famously said that a word only needed defining when it had come to misuse; this was what he observed to be happening in the 1940s around the word 'culture'. He noted at the time that the Oxford English Dictionary defined it as 'The setting of bounds; limitation'. The word predates the 1940s significantly but it has often been associated with ideals perceived to be different or unknown. Eighty years on and the scope of the word has broadened – there is less of a negative, fear association and more of a social norms and customs trend. Culture is something that should be celebrated as part of the make-up of a person's identity, whether it is something they are born into or are attracted to in adulthood.

Cultures have a multitude of elements but they all hold one thing in common – likeness amongst the people who make up a culture. This could be genetic, geographic, religious or linked with sexuality, or really anything across the biological, psychological or social spectrum. Everyone will hold a commonality but these will also not be specific or measurable. For example, everyone within the LGBTQ+ community holds a likeness of not following heterosexual relationship norms, but they will not all conform exclusively to singular same sex or gender relationships.

Those entering a culture in their teen years or early twenties, when identity is still developing, will bring with them a different cultural experience from childhood that will influence their identity. They will also find that their own relationship to their culture is dynamic and evolving, with how they choose to identify and present their needs as changeable. Acculturation may have occurred, where the person has moved away from one culture and adopted cultural traits from another, and therefore stereotypical expectations will differ. This is particularly prevalent amongst recent and hereditary migrants, who will have common cultural history but have adopted cultural elements from their new home. England is recognised to be a highly diverse country, with many subgroups from around the world. It is important to recognise that although they have come to live in this country, it is important to personal identity to maintain parts of their own culture.

Within working practice, the NA must ensure that they are inclusive and working in a diversity-positive way. This means advocating for patients' cultural needs and desires and being a role model to colleagues, making culture a prominent element in day-to-day care delivery. As professionals, we should also be challenging our own preconceived perceptions of how cultural variations present themselves.

Questions to Consider when Developing an Effective Nurse–Patient Relationship

As the welcoming healthcare professional, you may want to demonstrate your openness and knowledge of others. However, you also need to have realistic expectations about what knowledge you can retain on a variety of cultures – is it realistic to know every need and every adjustment, or is it instead reasonable to take the time to discuss their needs with the individual? As part of the data collection role of the NA, asking questions and being inquisitive confidently will not only ensure the person receives care that meets their needs, but it will make the person feel important and acknowledged as an individual. Taking the time to ask questions will build the therapeutic relationship.

A person's culture will have the potential to influence all areas of their lives, including their health choices, decisions and goals for recovery. Expect that when you ask questions, you may be exploring more than just their health, diet and faith needs.

- Language, dress, food, rituals, celebrations – easy to identify and simpler to address.
- Customs and rituals.
- Worship, religion and spiritual beliefs.
- Diet.
- Art and music.
- Humour.
- Education.
- Activity participation.
- Clothing, and attitudes towards cleanliness and formality.
- Hierarchy and gender roles.
- Upbringing and life experience.
- Expressing emotions, ethics, communication style, values, gender roles, privacy and modesty – need deeper collaboration and open discussion to ensure these needs are being met with respect.

Hall (1959) identified three main principles on which cultures differ: context, space and time. These principles are particularly relevant to receiving inpatient care, where the space and context – the hospital and being ill – significantly differ from when someone is living their normal life. The person will have a new level of need and reliance on others to meet their needs, and thus they may look upon their cultural needs differently. However, it is essential that they make those decisions and not the healthcare provider, and re-establish their cultural needs as they recover and see fit to follow these. For example, it is advised that if a person becomes unwell during Ramadan, they should stop fasting and seek healthcare support. It is then up to the person when they recommence fasting, and the healthcare professional's role is to respect this choice.

Barriers to Supporting Cultural Awareness

Your role will be to advocate this personal choice, and ensure consistent and up-to-date information is shared with others involved in the person's care. Advocating will also include challenging others' misconceptions of what culture means to your patients. The concept of cultural blindness is the claim to not see race, culture or ethnicity, and some may use this as a reference to treating everyone the same, and thus equally. However, one consequence of this is alienation and lack of thought to understand everyone as an individual. A person is less likely to seek out healthcare provision if they believe their cultural needs will be casually dismissed, rather than met.

It is not realistic to suggest that for every culture, you fully inform yourself of their needs. What is realistic is having awareness of the services that can provide support, such as chaplains and interpreters, and communicating with your patients sensitively around their needs.

Sensory and Altered Perceptions

A sensory or altered perception occurs when a person's reality and experience are different to those being observed by the wider community. This will be directly impacted by mental illness, learning difference, neurodiversity or chemical exposure. This could be thought of within the context of the Mental Capacity Assessment two-stage approach (Mental Capacity Act Code of Practice, p.41) as a diagnostically relevant impairment or disturbance in the functioning of their brain. This could be a temporary state, such as delirium, drug-induced psychosis or an acute onset of a known psychiatric illness. Or it could be a more chronic presentation such as dementia, learning disability or autism.

It is important in the context of mental capacity not to assume that just because a person has a relevant diagnosis, they will invariably have capacity over many elements of their lives, and assumptions must not be made about their ability to make decisions. Another key element to keep in mind is that although a diagnosis provides some scope for awareness to adapt communication, every person will present differently and therefore their communication needs will be different.

Recalling your preparation before the conversation, there are additional resources which may be available to these individuals. Utilising available information avoids repetition and frustration and is particularly valuable if you only have a short window of time to engage with your client and you need to make the most of that valuable time. Ideally, individuals with a learning disability will have a Communication Passport as part of their care plan, outlining their communication needs in a person-centred way, with positive focus on what the person can do, rather than what they cannot. This document will have similarities to the Advance Directives used in mental health services and the Respect forms used in end-of-life care.

Reflective Activity: Communication Passport

James is 25 years old and has arrived with his mum, Angela, to your department for a blood test. Angela presents you with his Communication Passport and asks you to help in making James' time in your department as comfortable as possible.

Important things you should know about me:

- *'I find it hard to understand long pieces of information'*

How I communicate:

- *'I enjoy talking, but when I am nervous or do not know you, I do not speak'*
- *'I will point at things, without making eye contact'*
- *'Please ignore me if I swear, I'm not angry, it's because I am anxious'*

Things I like:

■ *'Rugby, dogs, peanut butter, Xbox'*

Things I don't like:

■ *'Loud noises, strong smells, changes to my routine'*

Things you can do to help me:

■ *'Showing me the palms of your hands makes me feel more relaxed'*
■ *'Pointing to pictures from my folder as you are talking helps me remember what you have told me'*
■ *'Give me time to respond, sometimes I just need time to talk'*

Using ADPIE (see Chapter 3 for a reminder), plan how you would support James and his mum while meeting his communication needs.

Time is an important factor in communication, not just the amount but how it is used. It is also a known barrier to meaningful communication due to the competing pressures on time. However, if you are able to prioritise a conversation, it will save time in the long term and reduce distress, complications and potential errors.

If someone is experiencing disordered thinking or hallucinations, their ability to concentrate for an extended period may be affected but you do not necessarily need to set aside a large block of time; instead, planning small unobtrusive interactions without overwhelming questioning is key. You might also want to determine the best time of the day to interact with the individual. The term Sundowning® refers to the evening when service users with dementia may present as less cognitively aware of their surroundings, and therefore may be less able to engage in complex discussions or unwilling to talk. Choose a time when you have observed your service user to be more relaxed, willing to engage in small talk or at a set time following treatment.

The location of a conversation will always be an influential factor in the outcome. The obvious place has always been in a clinical room, as this sets the scene for the content of the conversation, but what does it say about the tone of the conversation? Cold, sterile, professional? Or do you want the conversation to be nurturing, supportive and collaborative? If so, and sterile clinical equipment is not a necessity, reconsider when you meet to talk. Ask the service user where they feel most comfortable; this may be a private space that they can talk freely without their thoughts being a barrier.

Location and time preferences do need to be weighed against risk for both of you. Is your clinic room going to cause distress and agitation or is their chosen environment an area you feel that you are unable to safely attend alone. Knowing and understanding the risks beforehand are essential, with risk being a multifaceted element.

Risk Factors

Risk to Self

Does the environment have objects that your service user could harm themselves on, or does the surrounding area and environment pose a risk by triggering past experiences or providing known opportunities to harm?

Risk to Others

Are they a particular threat to an identified gender "cultural group", or need more than one person in the room?

Risk from Others

Is there is a history of abuse, in which case they might not want to talk to someone who has similar identifiable features or struggle to be in an environment where they do not know how to escape.

Falls

Whether this is related to cognition, substance use or physical health, ensure the environment is safe for them to mobilise around.

Physical Causes of Communication Barriers

Although this might present as a very broad or vague title, the assessment of needs process will always start as follows; how long have you had this barrier, and to what extend does it impact on your communication needs?

For acute onset of a communication barrier, such as sudden hearing or vision loss, aphasia or delirium, the first action will be to establish what has caused this. This presentation may be part of a wider group of symptoms the person is exhibiting and ideally identifying and treating the cause will manage the communication barrier. At this point the communication barrier will either be resolved or it will move into the longer-term chronic stage.

An individual will have lived with chronic communication barriers for a non-determinant length of time, either from birth or acquired within their life, and managing an acute illness will not resolve the barrier. However, change to severity or additional new communication barriers may occur because of the acute illness. The communication barrier could also naturally worsen over time, as is the case with age-related hearing and vision loss.

The impact of a communication barrier on the person will depend on multiple factors that span the biological-psychological-social spectrum, and this historical impact will dictate how a person wants their needs to be met, or awareness of how their needs can be met.

Biological

- Number of barriers
- Severity of barrier

Psychological

- Isolation
- Neglect of needs
- Bullying based on needs
- Self-worth
- Self-consciousness

Social

- Schooling
- Access to learning multiple languages

Once you have established the long-term impact and severity of the barrier, you can prepare to make a plan with that individual for what they need. Hearing loss, for example, has a wide variation and to make assumptions about how someone can and wants to communicate will create additional barriers. For example, younger people may be more confident with sign language but may struggle with reading and writing, while someone with age-related hearing loss will be less likely to know sign language and may prefer written communication. Literacy levels within the deaf community are significantly below those of the hearing community (Herman et al. 2017). This is not a given and should not be assumed, but it is important that these options are considered.

You might also assume that someone can lip read as they have followed instructions but they may not feel confident to do this consistently, and it should not be assumed this is an acceptable way to aid communication. Similarly, hearing aids are not always appropriate, and if someone finds them uncomfortable or is self-conscious about them, they should not be forced onto the individual.

New onset or a change in someone's communication needs has a significant impact on mental health, due to isolation and frustration. Aphasia, for example, is linked to deterioration in social functioning, relationship development and poorer rehabilitation outcomes (Donnellan et al. 2010). If someone is feeling low in mood and struggling with feelings of reduced self-worth, their ability to engage openly and confidently with professionals about their care needs will be reduced. As an NA, you need to ensure that engagement with the person is consistent and instils feelings of worth in the person. You may be initiating conversations more frequently with that person but each interaction will build trust and therapeutic bonding, and together you will be able to explore what communication methods work best with them.

Tools used to communicate will vary depending on the circumstances, and thought should be given to availability of resources. Your service user's preference may be for a translator to be present, which would be necessary for important conversations and specific appointments but may not be realistic for 24-hour delivery. Therefore other methods that meet their needs, such as picture cards, may be utilised.

Distance communication, through written letters or over the phone, also presents barriers. Having clear documentation of choice of how that person wants to be contacted, whether that is via text message, through Braille or via their nominated advocate, is a necessary step to avoid discrimination.

Reflective Activity: Information for Service Users

Explore your working environment and look for any display or written information which is there for the attention of your service users. As you identify these, ask the followings questions.

- Are the instructions understandable?
- Are there words only a healthcare professional would understand?
- Are the colours clear?
- Could someone with a visual impairment read it?
- Is there guidance on how they could read it in a different format?

How can you ensure you working area is inclusive and meets all your service users' needs?

Resources such as objects and basic images which are readily available throughout your area, or on the internet, can be used as quick prompts to conversation, which when used with simple body language and facial expressions aid communication in the moment. The Mehrabian (1971) model of verbal and non-verbal communication notes that 55% of communication is in the body language, not words or tone, so extending the body to objects and images would boost this significant element of communication.

Challenging Conversations – Breaking Bad News and Emotionally Charged Situations

A challenging conversation would be considered one where you or the other members of the conversation may perceive the outcome to be contrary to their desired approach. However, this does not mean the course of the conversation will necessarily involve challenging each other.

A challenging conversation is very much influenced by your own personal experience and the emotions you bring to that situation. As discussed with experiential learning, if you have not previously been in a precise situation (telling a parent their child has cancer or a service user that their Mental Health Act Section has been upheld at tribunal), it is not possible for you to predict how you will carry out this conversation. And the same goes for that parent or service user – if the child has had cancer previously and the parent was aware that the symptoms were the same, they may have already expected the confirmation, and the service user may have been prepared by the care team and solicitor before the tribunal. The emotions that arise as the conversation progresses will influence how successfully the message is portrayed.

The perception of whether any conversation is negative or positive will also be influenced by experience. While you might believe your conversation is discussing a poor outcome, the client may feel relieved. As with the example of cancer, they may have been seeking answers for their symptoms for some time, and to know there is a definitive reason may be a relief. Therefore, predicting how a conversation will go is impossible, and instead preparation is necessary.

Preparation will come in the form of reflection. We have previously discussed reflection following situations and learning from them to improve future practice. This is an opportunity to bring that learning into action; before going into a difficult conversation, consider how you managed this last time, what went well, how did your emotions influence it, and how you can best manage this again. Without thorough reflection, you may only be carrying your emotions about the situation into your future practice, which in the case of challenging conversations are often emotions relating to fear, anxiety and sadness.

Your reflection may also lead to you considering your role within the conversation – are you the correct person to lead the conversation or do you have a different role to play? This will depend on your personal and professional experience and knowledge, your scope of practice and necessity for aftercare involvement. For some conversations, it is not about hierarchy, it will be dictated by therapeutic relationships and who the client feels more comfortable to meet with. Acknowledging how your emotions will influence how you carry out the conversation while reflecting is essential to ensure the client receives a focused and person-centred discussion – if you feel your emotions will affect this, then delegate the task to someone more appropriate.

It may have been decided that the conversation fits better in another professional's scope of practice but you are going to be part of the aftercare team, and being involved as an observer is necessary. Your role here would be providing ongoing reiteration of the information discussed and the plan made, ensuring that communication is accurate and provides reassurance. You will also observe how the client responds emotionally to the conversation, and ensure that all future conversation, whether delivered by yourself or another professional, reflects their emotional needs.

In order to aid a successful conversation, a model can be used to prepare and structure your conversation. The use of a model will not guarantee the outcome of a conversation but it will be a tool to aid your preparation and thus reduce any anxiety you may be experiencing.

SPIKES

The SPIKES acronym (Setting up, Perception, Invitation, Knowledge, Emotions, Strategy) is typically used when breaking bad news, whether that be a life-limiting or life-changing conversation. The model of Baile et al. (2000) was initially introduced within cancer care but the tool's simple six-step approach can be applicable to many different situations. As you read through the model and its instructions, consider how this would be useful in your clinical area, how much you feel you can manage and at what stages you would need support from others in preparation.

Setting Up the Interview

- *Rehearsal*: mentally planning what you are going to say and anticipating how the client may respond and the type of questions they may ask. You may want to prepare notes and have a pen and paper handy to record any questions they ask that you are unable to answer. This is your prompt to familiarise yourself with the options available to ensure the client can make well-informed decisions.
- *Environment*: the place you choose to have the conversation must be private, low stimulus and conducive to comfort. If you are restricted to a bay area, ensure the curtains are closed and an appropriate vocal volume is used to provide as much privacy as possible. Be prepared with tissues and a drink. Depending on the clinical area, you may be able to have hot drinks as well; a hot drink demonstrates your commitment to spend time talking with the person – you are inviting them to stay while the drink cools and they have time to drink it in comfort.
- *Advocate*: ensure they have someone with them to provide emotional support or advocate if they wish. This could be a family member, friend or appointed advocate or you might be that person.
- *Making connection*: maintaining rapport through empathy and active listening skills. Allowing them to express their feelings and engaging them in a conversation.
- *Time*: ensure you have set aside sufficient time to carry out your conversation; this also applies to interruptions.

Perception (Assessing the Patient's Perception)

'Before you tell, ask' (Baile et al. 2000). Using open questions, measure the client's perspective of what they understand so far, what they believe tests have been looking for and what they are expecting from this conversation. This will give you some idea of how they will react – either they already know there is a potential for bad news or they are unaware and have not had a chance to rationalise or plan for the potential worst.

Invitation (Obtaining the Patient Invitation)

Ask the client how much they want to know. Many people will want to know details so they can make plans and be prepared, but some will not be prepared to discuss all the details yet. This is a normal response as part of the grieving process and must be respected. This response may occur in all future appointments, or they may want more details after contemplation, so ensure you do not make assumptions at this stage even if you know the person.

Knowledge (Giving Knowledge and Information to the Patient)

This stage opens with the clear statement of direction of where the conversation is going: 'I am sorry to tell you...'. You may find that following this statement, your client will struggle to retain the information you are sharing due to their own thoughts; you will be able to go over the finer detail at later appointments, so make a note of what they have not followed. Ensure your language and any medical terminology used are appropriate to the individual's literacy level, checking understanding frequently. The temptation at this stage is to share everything you know without a pause, but this will leave the client overwhelmed and potentially frustrated, so regular check-ins of understanding are essential. Do not lie about improving the outcome – remain factual but compassionate.

*E*motions (Addressing the Patient's Emotions with Empathetic Responses)

- Emotions as well as understanding will dictate how much knowledge you impart to the client. If the client is visibly distressed, withdrawn or angry, allow them to feed back how they are feeling before continuing. They may also express feelings contrary to how you perceive the situation, such as relief or optimism – what you have told them might be the end of a long journey into an unknown future and instead of distress, they may be relieved to hear there is a plan.
- Acknowledging their emotions and encouraging them to discuss how they are feeling demonstrate an empathetic response and instil trust that you care for their journey. The range of emotions could potentially be wide at this stage and predicting them may be impossible, but whatever they express will be valid.

*S*trategy and Summary

- Before making or sharing a strategy, it is important to check with the client how they would like to go forward – have they already done some research or are they overwhelmed in this moment and not ready to discuss a plan? Ensure that the plan involves all the options either available through your service or wider. The client may have ideas which you deem to be unwise, and if this is the case ensure that they understand all the risks and benefits of this plan. If they have capacity, they have the right to make this decision.
- Summarising is the final opportunity in this meeting to confirm that the client has understood the discussion. Offer to provide them with a written summary of the meeting to take home with them, and appropriate contact details, and make a follow-up appointment to answer any new questions and review the plan. As the NA, this might be the stage where your role for ongoing support and source of knowledge is introduced, so be prepared to share your role and manage expectations.

Conflict and Challenging Behaviour

Emotional expression can come in many different forms, and it is important to acknowledge the expression of emotions such as anger and fear equally to happiness and excitement. But are you confident in observing and recognising signs of emotions?

Reflective Activity: Behavioural Manifestations

For each of the behaviours below, write a list or draw how that person will be presenting; what thoughts they will be having, what emotions they will be experiencing, and how their body will be responding. Use this as a chance to reflect on people you have delivered care to and how their behaviours have presented.

- Angry
- Excited
- Relaxed
- Anxious

This exercise is about the fight or flight response, where the person is not able to verbally tell you how they are feeling but through observation you can interpret their body language into emotions. Those presenting with anger or anxiety will exhibit very similar symptoms, as they will both be expressing the fight or flight signs.

Understanding the fight or flight response is key in managing conflict. The role of the professional is to recognise that there will always be a reason for conflict to occur, and rather than focusing on treating the symptoms of the behaviour, they should instead be identifying the causes and how to resolve those. Knowing someone's signs of escalation in advance is necessary to respond early; acknowledging this is their way of communicating their distress to you. Although hostility and aggression are socially unacceptable behaviours, they will arise when a need has not been met or recognised, which will in turn lead to frustration and then anger.

When displays of aggression are met with authority or resistance, the behaviour often escalates, so the more desired approach would be to avoid getting to that stage, but rather responding to early signs of emotional change. De-escalation techniques and conflict management use this method of early intervention to acknowledge emotions, listen to needs and provide open and honest support.

Active listening skills	Expected outcome
Using open-ended questions	Person gives more information
Providing encouragement	Person elaborates on topic
Paraphrasing statements	Person feels heard and validated
Reflecting of feelings	Person feels more understood
Summarising interaction	Person sees new meaning in their story

Avoid	Give	Explain	Commit
Avoid promising an unachievable solution	Give a range of realistic choices so the person can select what they believe will help	Explain what will be done, by whom and when	Commit to a realistic timeframe for the agreed course of action

Source: Adapted from Lowry (2016).

Conflict can also occur when two or more people envisage contradicting processes or outcomes from an event, each wishing to prioritise their own plan. This conflict can escalate with perceived communication techniques, listed below, which instead of supporting discussion can lead to blocking. Blocking behaviours deter communication and prevent the development of therapeutic rapport. If the patient perceives you to be exhibiting these behaviours, they will be reluctant to engage further or disclose problems for fear of not being listened to.

- *Offering advice and reassurance before the main problems have been identified*: the client might be reluctant to discuss what the root problem is for fear of causing offence, therefore the conflict remains unresolved.
- *Explaining away distress as normal*: emotions are normal, so encourage the expression of emotion. However, the distress and their perception attached to it is not normal, it is very personal. Suggesting it is normal will lead them to believe they have to respond the same as everyone else or that you are dismissing their concerns.
- *Attending to physical aspects only*: when delivering care, ensure you are taking a holistic approach as your view of the problem may differ from that of the client.
- *Switching the topic*: moving on before the client feels they are ready will result in them feeling dismissed and that their concerns are less important.
- *'Jollying' patients along*: this refers to rushing them. Ensure you have prepared time to engage on a more in-depth level.

Sometimes it is necessary to acknowledge that you may not be the right person to manage conflict. It may be that although you are a senior staff member, a more junior colleague has a better rapport with the person. You role instead will be to give your colleague support and guidance, and follow on the conversation once the situation has been de-escalated.

Application to Practice

When considering your clinical practice, understanding communication is essential, but even more important is your ability to autonomously apply the knowledge to your client's care. You may find yourself in the position of leading in many of the situations discussed in this chapter due to your holistic approach and broad experience, so preparation is key. Using a model such as the nursing process provides you with a structured approach through which you can meet the person's communication needs, and support in logically sharing your plan and justification for this with your colleagues.

The activity below provides a summary for the barriers discussed, but also gives you the opportunity to explore what resources you already have available to you in your practice, what you can implement and where additional training or education is needed for your team.

> **Reflective Activity: Planning Care for Effectively Managing Communication Barriers**
>
> Using ADPIE (see previous chapters), explore how you would meet these broad communication barriers.
>
> - Children
> - Culture
> - Sensory and altered perceptions
> - Hearing impairment
> - Challenging conversations

Professional and Team Communication

Professional communication is the use of communication within the working environment. This may be with patients and families, but it will also be with colleagues. The skills needed for professional communication will have been learned from the workplace; you will have observed how others communicate and unconsciously established which approaches form bonds, achieve goals and cause conflict. This is very much part of your development of self, as discussed at the start of the chapter. The skills you use with colleagues will be the same as those you use with patients, but you need to assess how much of your authentic self you will be comfortable to share and the situations in which you use your skills will be different.

The scenarios below reflect communication barriers that often present within healthcare – hierarchy, protecting your limitations and critical feedback. For each scenario, reflect on your own experience of how you have seen this managed previously, the emotions you experienced within this situation, and what you would need to confidently manage this yourself.

- A team member bypasses you for information on your patient to a more senior member of staff.
- You are asked to carry out a task you feel you have not had sufficient practice in and therefore feel unprepared for.
- A colleague has made an error in their documentation which you have observed and which requires escalation for correction.

Resources

The resources recommended within this chapter are not limited to specific communication barriers; they are multifunctional and can be used creatively by all to meet everyone's communication needs.

Social Stories are a tool initially introduced to support those with autism, but can also be easily used with children, those who do not read or speak English when interpreters are not available, and people with anxiety. Social Stories are a visual aid to guide the person on a picture-based journey of what they will be experiencing, for example going to a hospital appointment or getting ready in the morning. The tool is flexible, with images that can be specific photographs or clipart-style images, and words to a level that meets the client's reading skills. They can be used to either prompt memory of the plan or provide reassurance to alleviate anxiety and fear.

Dependent on the part you play in the person's care journey, you may not be involved in the formulation of the Social Story, but you may be asked to ensure it is available to the person when they are in your care, you may be asked to read with them regularly to familiarise them with the journey, or you may be contributing. In the role of advocate, you will be responsible for ensuring this story is available for the person, and that your colleagues and others involved in their care are utilising it.

Chapter Summary

This chapter has considered the complex and dynamic nature of effective communication and the necessity of ensuring that, as an NA, you have a well-developed sense of the importance of effective communication. The activities in this chapter have been suggested to support you to reflect and continually refine your communication skills as you progress within your role. This will help you to develop effective nurse–patient relationships so that you can effectively advocate and support your patient through well-considered communication strategies which meet individualised patient need.

References

Baile, W., Buckman, R., Lenzi, R. et al. (2000). SPIKES – a six-step protocol for delivering bad news; application to the patient with cancer. *Oncologist* 5 (4): 302–311.

Berlo, D.K. (1960). *The Process of Communication*. New York: Holt, Rinehart and Winston.

Bowlby, J. (1958). The nature of the child's tie to his mother. *International Journal of Psycho-analysis* 39: 350–373.

Cox, K. (2018). Use of emotional intelligence to enhance advanced practice registered nursing competencies. *Journal of Nursing Education* 57 (11): 648–654.

Cruess, R., Cruess, S., and Steinert, Y. (2016). *Teaching Medical Professionalism: Supporting the Development of the Professional Identity*. Cambridge: Cambridge University Press.

Danieli, Y. (1998). *International Handbook of Multigenerational Legacies of Trauma*. Boston: Springer.

Donnellan, C., Hickey, A., Hevey, D.a., and O'Neill, D. (2010). Effect of mood symptoms on recovery one year after stroke. *International Journal of Geriatric Psychiatry* 25 (12): 1288–1295.

Giroux, H. and Penna, A. (1983). Social education in the classroom; the dynamic of the hidden curriculum. In: *The Hidden Curriculum and Moral Education* (ed. H. Giroux and D. Purpel). San Francisco: McCutchan Publishing Corporation.

Hall, E.T. (1959). *The Silent Language*. New York: Doubleday.

Hall, E. (1966). *The Hidden Dimensions*. New York: Anchor Books.

Herman, R. Roy, P. and Kyle, F. (2017). Reading and Dyslexia in Deaf Children. www.city.ac.uk/__data/assets/pdf_file/0005/564170/Reading–and–Dyslexia-in-Deaf-Children-Herman-Roy-Kyle-2017-FINAL.pdf

Heron, J. (2001). *Helping the Client: A Creative Practical Guide*, 5e. London: Sage.

Lowry, M. (2016). Deescalating anger: a new model for practice. *Nursing Times* 112 (4): 4–7.

Maguire, P.a. and Pitceathly, C. (2002). Key communication skills and how to acquire them. *BMJ* 325: 697–700.

Malviya, S., Voepel-Lewis, T., Burke, C. et al. (2006). The revised FLACC observational pain tool: improved reliability and validity for pain assessment in children with cognitive impairment. *Paediatric Anaesthetics* 16 (3): 258–265.

Mehrabian, A. (1971). *Silent Messages*. Belmont: Wadsworth.

Miller, W. and Rollnick, S. (2012). *Motivational Interviewing*, 3e. New York: Guilford Press.

Nursing and Midwifery Council (NMC) (2018). *Standards of Proficiency for Nurses, Midwives and Nursing Associates*. London: Nursing and Midwifery Council.

Peplau, H.E. (1991). *Interpersonal Relations in Nursing: A Conceptual Framework of Reference for Psychodynamic Nursing*. New York: Springer.

Salovey, P.a. and Mayer, J. (1990). Emotional intelligence. *Imagination, Cognition and Personality* 9 (3): 185–211.

Shannon, C. and Weaver, W. (1949). *The Mathematical Theory of Communication*. Chicago: University of Illinois Press.

Stead, B.A. (1972). Berlo's communication process model as applied to the behavioural theories of Maslow, Herzberg and McGregor. *Academy of Management Journal* 15 (3): 389–394.

Stewart, D., Burrow, H., Duckworth, A. et al. (2015). Thematic analysis of psychiatric patients' perceptions of nursing staff. *International Journal of Mental Health Nursing* 1 (24): 82–90.

Woodbridge, K.a. and Fulford, B. (2004). Right, wrong and respect. *Mental Health Today* Sep: 28–30.

Further Reading

Blackburn, C. and Harvey, M. (2018). A different kind of normal: parents' experiences of early care and education for young children born prematurely. *Early Child Development and Care* 190 (3): 296–309.

Cherniss, C. (2010). Emotional intelligence: towards clarification of a concept. *Industrial and Organizational Psychology* 3 (2): 110–126.

Eliot, T.S. (1948). *Notes Towards the Definition of Culture*. London: Faber and Faber.

Fulford, K.W.M. (2004). *Whose Values? A Workbook for Values-Based Practice in Mental Health Care* (ed. K. Woodbridge). London: Sainsbury Centre for Mental Health.

Handelzalts, J., Levy, S., Molmen-Lichter, M. et al. (2021). The association of attachment style, postpartum PTSD and depression with bonding – a longitudinal path analysis model, from childbirth to six months. *Journal of Affective Disorders* 280: 17–25.

Holmes, J. (2014). *John Bowlby and Attachment Theory*. London: Routledge.

Murray, R.a. and Dunn, S. (2017). Assessing nurses' knowledge of spiritual care practices before and after an educational workshop. *Journal of Continuing Education in Nursing* 48 (3): 115–122.

Nelson, H. (2024). Experiencing birth trauma: individualism and isolation in postpartum. *Social Science and Medicine* 345: 116663.

Paris, J. (2020). *Nature and Nurture in Mental Disorders: A Gene–Environment Model*. Washington DC: America Psychiatric Association Publishing.

6

The Nursing Associate and Duty of Care, Candour, Equality and Diversity

Marie Knight

University Hospitals of Leicester NHS Trust, Leicester, UK

Introduction

Duty of care, candour and equality and diversity are concepts that are often discussed when considering nursing and keeping our patients safe but what do they really mean? This chapter will explore these three concepts in more detail, how they interlink and their relevance to you as a nursing associate (NA).

While there is a common understanding that we have a duty of care when asked, this is hard to define and the lack of underpinning evidence makes this more challenging. The literature to support this is lacking and there is very little evidence to demonstrate what feels like a vital core to the profession of both nursing and healthcare.

Aims of This Chapter

- Consider the relevance and importance of the duty of care and explore ways in which reasonable care can be taken to avoid acts or omissions which might reasonably be foreseen as likely to cause harm.
- Explore the relevance and significance of duty of candour and examine the ways in which this can and should be demonstrated in practice.
- Reflect on why basic rights and principles of dignity, equality, diversity, humanity and safeguarding are important across a range of health and care settings to identify when people may need help to facilitate equitable access to care.

The Nursing Associate: Stepping into Practice, First Edition. Edited by Annabel Coulson.
© 2025 John Wiley & Sons Ltd. Published 2025 by John Wiley & Sons Ltd.

Related NMC Standards

- ▪ 2.4 Understand the factors that may lead to inequalities in health outcomes.
- ▪ 2.6 Understand and explain the contribution of social influences, health literacy, individual circumstances, behaviours, and lifestyle choices to mental, physical and behavioural health outcomes.
- ▪ 3.21 Recognise how a person's capacity affects their ability to make decisions about their own care and to give or withhold consent.
- ▪ 3.22 Recognise when capacity has changed and understand where and how to seek guidance and support from others to ensure that the best interests of those receiving care are upheld.

Duty of Care

Nursing is a profession rooted in compassion, expertise and a profound commitment to the wellbeing of others. At the heart of nursing practice lies the concept of duty of care, which underpins various aspects of society from healthcare to business, to everyday interactions. At its core, duty of care refers to the legal and ethical obligation to act in a manner that avoids causing harm to others. It is a principle deeply rooted in moral philosophy and is often seen as the cornerstone of responsible behaviour.

There has also been an established recognition in the courts that nurses and NAs owe a duty of care to their patients (Griffith 2014) The NMC Code (2018) is less prescriptive but despite it alluding to nurses and NAs having a duty of care, it does not specifically direct this. The Code considers the need to treat people as individuals and states the following under the Prioritising People section.

Prioritise People

> *You put the interests of people using or needing nursing or midwifery services first. You make their care and safety your main concern and make sure that their dignity is preserved, and their needs are recognised, assessed and responded to. You make sure that those receiving care are treated with respect, that their rights are upheld and that any discriminatory attitudes and behaviours towards those receiving care are challenged.*

Treat people as individuals and uphold their dignity
To achieve this, you must:

1.1 treat people with kindness, respect and compassion.

1.2 make sure you deliver the fundamentals of care effectively.

1.3 avoid making assumptions and recognise diversity and individual choice.

1.4 make sure that any treatment, assistance or care for which you are responsible is delivered without undue delay.

1.5 respect and uphold people's human rights (NMC 2018).

While this may be helpful, it does not explain fully what our duty of care to our patients is and some of the terminology can be seen to provide overarching guidance but not what NAs should do. The Code further explores tasks such as maintaining hygiene and supporting patients to eat and drink who are not able to feed themselves but there remains a lack of clarity as to what duty of care means. This could lead the duty of care to be mistaken for the 'tasks' that are carried out; for example, the recording of a patient's blood pressure rather than the overarching duty of care of keeping our patients safe which can arguably be more difficult to define.

The introduction of the Human rights Act 1998 obligated the government to enact laws to confirm that the safety of patients is maintained by ensuring that nursing staff along with others do not violate an individual's rights. This is particularly important as many of our patients are vulnerable, which means that we need to act in their best interests and challenge care that we feel is inadequate. This is an important role for the registered nurse (RN) and NA and as a newly registered NA this can feel daunting, and you may need support to learn the skills of challenging any poor practice that may seem to be accepted within a workplace culture (Benner 1984).

As an NA, you are a crucial member of the healthcare team, providing essential support to RNs and the wider multidisciplinary team (MDT). NAs have a responsibility to ensure the safety and wellbeing of patients under their care. This includes following recognised protocols for administering medications, assisting with procedures and monitoring patients for any signs of deterioration.

Historically there have been instances where duty of care was not managed well, such as the case of Elizabeth Dixon, a young child who died because of multiple factors including a lack of communication in the form of both written and verbal handovers. There were missed opportunities to put safeguarding measures in place, and what could be considered hostile responses from some healthcare professionals, identified in the exploration and legal investigation into the death of Elizabeth. It took 20 years of the family fighting for answers to their questions in relation to the death of their daughter to identify lessons to be learnt. This also made it clear that to provide safe effective care to our patients, we need to consider any omissions or gaps in the care we provide as the omissions can have a significant impact on patient safety. Read more about Elizabeth Dixon here: www.gov.uk/government/publications/the-life-and-death-of-elizabeth-dixon-a-catalyst-for-change

Duty of care is underpinned by several key factors.

Professional Competence

As an NA, you must maintain a high level of competence in your practice (NMC 2018). This involves staying up to date with relevant training and education, adhering to professional standards and guidelines, and seeking assistance or clarification when faced with unfamiliar situations. The importance of this was highlighted by the Francis Report where there were systemic failings and neglect in the care of patients (Francis 2013).

Effective Communication

Effective communication is essential for fulfilling your duty of care, as it allows individuals to convey important information, seek consent and address concerns in a timely manner. This includes providing clear and accurate instructions, disclosing relevant risks and encouraging open conversation with patients, families or other professionals. Transparency fosters trust and enables collaborative decision making, ultimately promoting better outcomes for all, enhancing quality care. NAs must communicate clearly and effectively to ensure that information is accurately conveyed and understood.

Communication is integral to the work of an NA and plays a considerable part in the development of the nurse–patient relationship. It may be thought that if a patient is unable to speak, they are unable to communicate but this could not be further from the truth. A smile, a facial expression or a sound can all contribute to communication. Any negative behaviour of your patient, particularly those who cannot communicate verbally, is an equally valid although often less welcome form of communication (see Chapter 5 for an in-depth look at the importance of communication).

Advocacy

Nursing associates serve as advocates for their patients, ensuring that their needs and preferences are respected and addressed (NMC 2018). This may involve speaking up on behalf of patients who are unable to advocate for themselves, ensuring that their views and perspectives are upheld and their voices are heard. By empowering patients to actively participate in their healthcare decisions and advocating for their needs, NAs uphold their duty of care and promote patient-centred care delivery. Advocacy is an essential skill for a NA, particularly for those patients who may not be able to speak up for themselves for a range of reasons such as language, poor health literacy, those lacking in confidence or who may have mental health issues, impaired cognitive understanding or mental capacity.

Understanding the Mental Capacity Act (2005) is vital to ensure that patients have their needs met appropriately. The patient's wishes need to be considered as well as those of their relatives and carers, if appropriate. For those patients considered to have mental capacity, their consent needs to be sought prior to discussing their care with their relatives.

As an NA, assessing mental capacity can seem daunting and for some patients this assessment can be complex. It is important to understand that while you can carry out mental capacity assessments on things that are straightforward, such as consent to support with hygiene needs following incontinence, more complex assessments would not be carried out in isolation from the MDT. The appropriate professional needs to carry out the assessment; for example, if the patient needs a surgical procedure, then a surgeon has to complete the assessment as they can give the detail the patient needs to ensure the patient is able to give informed consent.

One of the overarching elements of consent is that the patient can change their mind, and can withdraw consent at any point. The primary principles of consent are that it must be voluntary and informed, and the patient must be capable of giving consent.

Ethical Practice

As an NA, you must adhere to ethical principles in your practice, including respect for patient autonomy, confidentiality and honesty (NMC 2018). You will be expected to navigate complex ethical dilemmas with integrity and professionalism, always prioritising the best interests of your patients. Sometimes you might face tough choices or situations where what is best for one patient might not be best for another. In these circumstances you may want to ask the RN to support the patient with decision making if you feel this is outside your scope of practice or expertise (see Chapter 3 for more detail on the importance of scope of practice).

Overall, duty of care in nursing is inseparable from ethical principles and values, guiding RNs and NAs in their commitment to providing safe, compassionate and ethical care to patients while upholding the highest standards of professionalism and integrity.

Continuous Improvement

As an NA, you should engage in ongoing reflection and self-assessment to identify areas for improvement in your practice (NMC 2018) You should actively seek feedback from colleagues and supervisors and participate in professional development activities, such as clinical supervision, to enhance your knowledge and skills.

In the UK, the NMC is the regulatory body responsible for setting standards for education, training, practice and the conduct for nurses, midwives and nursing associates. The NMC does this by regulating NAs and ensuring that they meet the necessary standard of competence to practise safely and effectively. As an NA, you must be registered with the NMC to work legally in the UK. The NMC requires NAs to engage in continuing professional development (CPD) and complete revalidation to maintain registration with the NMC. Overall, the NMC plays a central role in ensuring the quality, safety and professionalism of nursing practice in the UK. Continuous improvement and duty of care are interconnected concepts in nursing, both focusing on enhancing patient outcomes and ensuring the provision of safe, effective and compassionate care.

When thinking about your duty of care towards your patients, it is important to consider the physical, emotional and psychological care they receive. This is influenced by a multitude of factors, including staffing levels, time and financial restrictions alongside historical practices and workplace culture. While recognising that there must be some structure to healthcare to facilitate effective functioning and to meet patient need, for example protected mealtimes and standardised medication times, there also must be some flexibility to prevent the adverse impacts of institutional care. If you are working in a community setting, you will be aware that you are a visitor within the patient's home and as such there is a heavy reliance on negotiation and information giving to obtain consent and support compliance with healthcare. However, for those of you within the hospital or in residential settings, there may be an overreliance on historical ways of practising and a resistance to challenge the status quo. As an NA, you can question whether these practices are always in the best interests of the patient. It can be difficult to challenge accepted practice so gaining support from the RN will help you in the development of these skills.

Challenging poor practice and the receptiveness of the organisation to change are influenced by the responses to whistleblowing, suggestions from staff or patients and carers and progressive discussions. It is important to consider whether there are further areas where more flexible working may improve the care received by patients. These may include things such as reviewing the skill mix of staff on duty or a flexible working pattern for staff. As an NA, there are areas where you can influence change; this may be something as simple as considering the way information is communicated to the patient. Improved ways of working and governance have arisen in response to the findings in the Francis Report, and this has had a significant impact in policy making, improving practice, standardising and monitoring the care received (Francis 2013).

It is recognised that staffing levels are not always optimal. The UK government has resisted highlighting what minimal staffing levels should be, so although levels are suggested, they are not mandated. There is no accepted ratio of temporary staff to substantive staff; increased use of temporary staff can significantly affect the continuity and arguably the quality of care the patient receives. It has been recognised by numerous research studies that the higher the RN staff numbers, the lower the rates of death and infections (Mwansa Nkowane and Ferguson 2016). Also, higher levels of registered staff caring for patients directly correlate to an improvement in patient safety and subsequent quality of care. The NMC (2023) highlights that the number of NAs on the register is increasing, from 489 NAs in 2019 to more than 10,000 in 2023. It is hoped that this development is driven by a desire to increase patient' safety and it is anticipated that the numbers of NAs will increase.

While you should always try to include your patients in their care, there are times when the care for patients cannot be negotiated and discussed in the usual way and decisions may need to be taken for patients in their best interests. An example of this would be patients admitted to an emergency department following major trauma, or those who have impaired capacity due to illness or intoxication. This leads to a greater responsibility falling to the health professionals, and in turn means that the overarching duty of care becomes more complex and arguably more important.

Monitoring of duty of care has historically been managed in the courts using the Bolam test to assess if the duty of care has been applied (Bolam 1957). The Bolam test is a legal principle established in English law through the landmark case Bolam v Friern Hospital Management Committee in 1957. This case set a precedent regarding the standard of care expected from healthcare professionals, particularly in the context of medical negligence claims. The Bolam test states that the healthcare professional will not be considered negligent if they act in accordance with a practice accepted by a responsible body of medical professionals skilled in that field, even if there are differing opinions within the medical community.

However, the Bolam test has been subject to criticism and refinement over time. Subsequent legal cases, such as Bolitho v City and Hackney Health Authority in 1998, introduced the concept that the court can assess whether the medical opinion relied upon is logically defensible. Even if a practice is widely accepted within a medical community, it may still be considered negligent if it cannot be supported by logical reasoning or evidence. For NAs, this would apply if those who are considered to have breached duty of care following local investigation are referred to a NMC Fitness to Practise Panel. The Panel would determine whether there was any breach in the duty of care (NMC 2018).

Duty of Candour

While there is much written around 'duty of candour', the vast majority is concerned with 'when things go wrong', with many legal cases suggesting that as healthcare professionals, we do not always get things right. However, duty of candour covers more than this and is about having ongoing open and honest conversations with our patients and their relatives, while also allowing, encouraging and facilitating staff to raise their concerns. Creating a workplace culture where staff feel able to bring contributions to the development of the service is essential. It is equally important that any concerns are listened to and acted on appropriately. This has previously been negatively evidenced by the media who have reported on the regular investigations into healthcare trusts where care has failed but healthcare whistleblowing has been evident but not responded to positively.

The provision of person-centred care creates a unique position whereby difficult decisions may need to be made which do not satisfy all parties involved. For example, there may be instances where prognosis is poor such as when brain activity is not detected in ventilated patients, but from a relative's perspective the patient is still breathing so therefore is still alive. While this is not related to an error in care, the duty of candour principles are just as important, and this can be distressing for the patient or relative and for the members of staff.

Duty of candour is a difficult concept for students to understand, particularly in relation to open and honest conversations with patients and their families in more day-to-day situations, and they find it much easier to understand in relation to when mistakes have occurred. NAs need to understand the concept of duty of candour as an integral aspect of their day-to-day communication, as well as recognising its importance during difficult conversations necessary regarding ongoing treatment and personal wishes during the final stages of life. It is about helping you as an NA to develop the autonomy, confidence and authority to have appropriate conversations without automatic deferral to senior staff, but recognising and acting when wishes or issues need to be escalated (NMC 2018).

As an NA, you may be involved in situations where the duty of candour principle is paramount in the delivery of person-centred care. Seeking support and advice from the RN is important while you are also actively involved in taking a lead role in these situations in order to grow within the role.

Examples of the application of 'duty of candour' include the following.

Disclosure of Adverse Events

Nurses and NAs are obligated to disclose adverse events or incidents to patients and their families in a timely manner. This involves providing a clear and honest explanation of what happened, expressing empathy for any harm caused and discussing plans for follow-up care or resolution. This is not necessarily in the context of significant harm events but could be something as simple as a delay in passing on telephoned messages due to the needs of an unwell patient.

Supporting the Patient

As an NA, your role in the duty of candour includes providing vital support to patients and their families during difficult situations. You should offer emotional support and answer questions to the best of your ability, within your scope of practice, escalating to RNs and the appropriate MDT member as appropriate.

Documentation and Reporting

As an NA, you are responsible for accurately documenting all aspects of patient care, including conversations had in relation to healthcare planned and delivered.

You will need to be non-judgemental and recognise when people express wishes which may not reflect your own moral or personal values; you need to acknowledge that values held by both the patient and the NA are of equal validity, assuming that they are both legal and fulfil the criteria established in the Mental Capacity Act 2005. You need to recognise and understand the values and wishes the patient holds; patients who can communicate may be able to express these themselves. You need to ensure that patients are given the necessary opportunities and settings to express their views and you may need to explore alternative ways of enabling the less able patient to make their wishes understood. To facilitate this, reasonable adjustments may need to be made and can include the organisation of approved interpreters if needed to support individuals to make key decisions in their care. For some individuals, this will require you to allow time and a quiet space to process the information. Facilitating communication in alternative ways also needs to be explored, such as by writing, non-verbal communication, picture books or involvement of other MDT members who can offer support, for example speech and language therapists, occupational therapists or chaplaincy services.

Family and friends may also be involved in decision making but only with the patient's consent. Caution is required in this situation, particularly if the patient has impaired capacity or cannot consent and we need to act in their best interests. While recognising that the vast majority of friends and family would want to uphold the wishes of their loved ones, it needs to be borne in mind that some may not agree with the patient's wishes, as there may be some internal conflict or indeed an alternative agenda that makes decision making on behalf of the patient more complex.

Mental Capacity

If it has been established, through appropriate assessment, that the patient lacks mental capacity, this further complicates decisions that need to be made. One of the factors that needs to be considered is whether the patient is likely to regain capacity; for example, when a patient needs treating with antibiotics for an infection, loss of capacity should be time limited. In this instance, the issue is whether the decision needs to be made today or whether delaying the decision would be safe to allow the patient to make their own informed choice. It is also important to bear in mind that while a patient may not have mental capacity for a specific issue regarding treatment, they still have the right and potential capacity to make other decisions in relation to their care. For example, they may not have capacity to make complex decisions such as consent for surgery but could decide on the smaller parts of day-to-day care such as what to eat, drink or wear or whether to have their blood pressure taken, so it is important to always keep in mind that mental capacity is very much decision specific.

Patients may already have made their wishes known regarding certain circumstances, through advance decision documents, by use of a Respect form or lasting power of attorney. They may have discussed certain situations with next of kin or family but this is not necessarily the case, and they may have either changed their minds since those discussions or had documents completed.

It seems to be a commonly held belief that mental capacity is assessed by medical staff, and while this may be the case for complex care, as an NA you need to recognise that you are informally assessing patients' mental capacity every day.

For a formal capacity assessment, there are five guiding principles set out in the Mental Capacity Act 2005 (Section 2).

1. A person must be assumed to have capacity unless it is deemed that they do not have capacity.
2. Take all practicable steps to enable someone to make the decision.
3. People are allowed to make unwise decisions.
4. The least restrictive alternative should be identified if required.
5. If someone is found not to have mental capacity, you must act in their best interests.

The two-stage test for mental capacity starts with the diagnostic test, which requires the person to have a disturbance in the functioning of the mind or brain. The second stage is the functional test which assesses the following.

- Can the individual understand all the relevant information?
- Can the individual retain the information long enough to make the decision?
- Can the individual use or weigh the information as part of a process to arrive at a decision?
- Can the individual communicate the decision?

The recognition that not all patients have mental capacity, and that this may be fluctuating, is just as crucial for NAs as it is for RNs. NAs have a responsibility to communicate openly and honestly with patients, their families and other members of the healthcare team. This includes not only being transparent about care provided but also when having 'difficult conversations'.

Reflective Activity: Difficult Conversations

Think of a time within your practice when you had to have a difficult conversation with a patient. For example, there may have been an occasion where there was 'bad news' to be given or the expectations of the patient may not have been possible.

- How did you manage this situation?
- Did you need to escalate this?
- Would you do things differently if you encountered this situation again?

While recognising that duty of candour is more complex than just 'when things go wrong', these are often the most stressful situations for you as the NA, not least because most of the time you will have been trying your hardest to get things right. In these situations, there need to be opportunities for you to discuss your reaction to this and be supported; examples of this may include clinical supervision, critical incident debriefing sessions or Freedom to Speak Up guardians. As an NA, you may be involved in quite stressful or potentially confrontational discussions, even if only as a first point of contact which you then either deal with or escalate. If you need support or advice following these conversations, it is important that you know there is support specifically for these events, so you are not the odd one out, and that help is available. Your manager would normally be a good first point of contact.

Equality and Diversity

The concept of equality and diversity is concerned with treating people equitably, so allowing the population the same opportunities to achieve the same health outcomes.

Over the past 20 years in the UK, there has been a change in the population diversity which will have an impact on the care our developing patient group will need. The changing picture of our ethnically diverse population is captured in Table 6.1.

Table 6.1 highlights the changes in ethnic populations but the local picture may look very different from this. Ensuring the local healthcare service is accessible and meeting the needs of everyone is a challenge that all

Table 6.1: Changes in UK ethnicity over the last 20 years.

Ethnicity	2021	2011	2001
Asian	9.3%	7.5%	4.4%
Black	4.0%	3.3%	2.2%
Mixed	2.9%	2.2%	1.3%
White	81.7%	86%	91.3%
Other	2.1%	1.0%	0.9%

Source: Office for National Statistics (2021).

healthcare workers need to embrace as populations may have very different needs. This is supported by the Equality Act (2010) which gives guidelines on offering support to all our patients to ensure they understand their care, are able to participate in it and make choices that mean they receive the healthcare they need. Some patients will find this straightforward but for others it may be more complex and require more help from the NA as well as their friends and family.

The misconception that equality and diversity is about offering the same service to everyone will not be enough to meet the needs of our patients. By treating people equally, we are simply offering all our patients the same opportunities. This is unlikely to be enough to ensure that all patients can access the services we offer so we need to think about how we can support all our patients to receive the same treatment outcomes. For example, during the COVID-19 pandemic, the UK government organised for people to go house to house, ensuring their representatives were able to speak the same language as the high-risk communities who may not have had access to or understanding of the risks and benefits of accepting COVID-19 vaccinations.

Under the Equality Act it is law that we *make 'reasonable adjustments' for* our patients. This may be as simple as providing a quiet area for conversation to happen, offering translation services or allowing more time for understanding and the opportunities for questions. While we may need to supply high-quality information in different languages or font sizes, or provide opportunities for individual discussions with a pharmacist regarding the components of medication, or a multiprofessional meeting with interpreting services, we should not assume these measures will be sufficient.

Reflective Activity: Adjustments

Thinking about the area you work in, consider a time when a reasonable adjustment was made that had a positive impact on patient care. Now consider when a reasonable adjustment was not made but could/should have been – what were the implications of this? How could you as a NA support changes to further improve the equality and diversity aspects of care in your area?

Another area that needs to be considered within healthcare is the jargon and acronyms used which don't help the patient to understand what is being said and can also lead to misunderstandings amongst healthcare professionals. Working in more specialised areas has a unique benefit for the patient but it can mean that we almost talk in our own language. This is obvious when you first start in a new area and if you are struggling to understand, it must be almost impossible for some of our patients.

Complex medical terminology or jargon can hinder understanding during difficult conversations. Healthcare professionals should use plain language and avoid technical terms, ensuring that the information is easily understood. The NA plays a unique role in this as you are 'by the bedside' and can often build more meaningful relationships with patients so you are in a position to identify difficulties in fully understanding issues discussed.

It is important to recognise that along with this, patients will have different levels of understanding; this is known as health literacy. Health literacy is an important aspect to consider when looking at duty of care and candour. It also has an important role in aiming to support the equality and diversity needs of our patients. Not only do we need to consider the verbal language of the patient but also whether they can read this language or have a different regional dialect to the one used in the patient information leaflet, whether the medical terminology is translatable, and whether people can understand the information provided to make an informed decision.

It is recognised that approximately 20% of the population may not be able to read and/or understand the written information we give to them, and this increases in the older population, particularly for those who have long-term conditions, where it is important that they understand treatment options often for multiple co-morbidities. We so often default to giving patients written information without considering whether the patient can read it and as NAs, we should be checking that the patient is able to understand the information we are giving them, being aware that this is not automatically the case.

We also need to consider cultural and religious norms and requirements. For example, patients may consider some surgical procedures or ingredients in medication to be inappropriate for their cultural beliefs. NAs can promote the health literacy of our patients and you need to be aware of the range of services available within your area to facilitate patients to make an informed choice. These may include services such as translation and advocacy services, including Patient Advice and Liaison Services.

Chapter Summary

Nursing associates play a critical role in duty of care and candour in healthcare practice. By fostering open communication, providing support to patients and families, and collaborating with the healthcare team, NAs contribute to a culture of transparency, trust and patient-centred care. While duty of care, candour and equality and diversity have been discussed as separate concepts, it is important to recognise that these three cornerstones to care are interdependent and integral throughout the patient's healthcare journey. It can be difficult to separate out the concepts due to the interdependent relationships, particularly the duty of candour aspect, and this may possibly reflect the abundance of literature in relation to when things go wrong at the expense of exploring how this can and should be used in everyday situations. These theories allow the NA the opportunity for further exploration of these themes to be able to use the theory and examples to improve the quality and effectiveness of their practice.

References

Benner, P. (1984). From novice to expert, excellence and power in clinical nursing practice. *Research in Nursing & Health* 8 (1): 95–97.

Bolam v Friern Hospital Management Committee (1957). 1 WLR 583 www. healthcareethicsandlaw.co.uk/negligence-1/bolam-v-friern-hospital-management-committee-1957-bolam-test

Equality Act (2010). www.legislation.gov.uk/ukpga/2010/15/contents

Francis, R. (2013). *Report of the Mid Staffordshire NHS Trust Public Inquiry – Executive Summary*. London: Stationery Office.

Griffith, R. (2014). Duty of care is underpinned by a range of obligations. *British Journal of Nursing* 23 (4): 234–235.

Mental Capacity Act (2005). www.legislation.gov.uk/ukpga/2005/9/contents

Mwansa Nkowane, A. and Ferguson, S. (2016). The World Health Organization launches the 2016–2020 global strategic directions for strengthening nursing and midwifery. *Nursing Economics* 34 (4): 206–207.

Nursing and Midwifery Council (NMC) (2018). The Code: Professional Standards of Practice and Behaviour for Nurses, Midwives and Nursing Associates. www.nmc.org.uk/globalassets/sitedocuments/nmc-publications/nmc-code.pdf

Nursing and Midwifery Council (NMC) (2023). Registration data reports. www.nmc.org.uk/about-us/reports-and-accounts/registration-statistics

Office for National Statistics (2021). www.ethnicity-facts-figures.service.gov.uk/uk-population-by-ethnicity/national-and-regional-populations/population-of-england-and-wales/latest/#by-ethnicity-over-time-5-groups

Further Reading

Dowie, I. (2017). Legal, ethical and professional aspects of duty of care for nurses. *Nursing Standard* 32 (16–19): 47–52.

Griffiths, P., Recio-Saucedo, A., Dall'Ora, C. et al. (2018). The association between nurse staffing and omissions in nursing care: a systematic review. *Journal of Advanced Nursing* 74 (7): 1474–1487.

World Health Organization (2016). Global strategic directions for strengthening nursing and midwifery 2016–2020. https://iris.who.int/bitstream/handle/10665/275453/9789241510455-eng.pdf

7

The Team Around the Patient

Colette Orton

University Hospitals of Leicester NHS Trust, Leicester, UK

Introduction

This chapter will explore what teamwork and collaborative practice are and how healthcare professionals can deliver safe care and contribute to continuous improvement in services. Nursing associates (NA), by the nature of the role, are ideally placed to deliver and improve care, monitor patient conditions and promote patient safety. They play an important part as members of interdisciplinary teams, collaborating and communicating effectively with nurses, a range of other health and care professionals and lay carers (NMC Platform 4). Nursing associates improve the quality of care by contributing to the continuous monitoring of people's experience of care. They identify risks to safety or experience and take appropriate action, putting the best interests, needs and preferences of people first (NMC Platform 5).

This chapter focuses on themes that are inextricably linked to teamwork and collaborative practice. These include communication and in particular the way in which digital technology is being used increasingly in healthcare. There will be a review of what critical thinking is and the role it plays in supporting problem solving, decision making and the prioritisation of tasks. Linked to this are the topics of accountability, delegation and assertiveness. The inclusion of human and environmental factors, what they are and their influence on patient and staff safety will support the wider discussion on team working and collaborative practice. We willl review the individual roles of members of the interdisciplinary team, with an emphasis on the NA role. Understanding individual roles is imperative in terms of collaboration and delivering safe patient care. Culture is therefore central to discussions about teamwork. We also include here the importance of psychological safety and learning environments in terms of developing a positive culture that focuses on learning, improvements and patient safety. As leadership is at the forefront of teamwork, there will be

The Nursing Associate: Stepping into Practice, First Edition. Edited by Annabel Coulson.
© 2025 John Wiley & Sons Ltd. Published 2025 by John Wiley & Sons Ltd.

an overview of theories and styles of leadership. This will cover the role that the NA plays in care delivery and when they are involved in innovations in care.

Aims of the Chapter

To understand:

- the role of the NA in improving care and patient safety outcomes
- teamwork and collaborative practice to improve safety
- factors that contribute to and impact on patient safety – human and environmental factors, health and safety and risk assessment
- improving services, innovation and change
- leadership and patient safety.

Related NMC Standards

Platforms 3 and 4 are discussed throughout this chapter.

Teams

It is implicit that the patient is at the centre of what healthcare professionals do. Therefore, the patient is the most important person in any team.

The landscape of healthcare is constantly changing (Walsh and de Sarandy 2023). The shifting demographic of the population along with their presentations of complex conditions and multiple co-morbidities all place additional demands on the team around the patient.

Teams are dynamic and diverse and it is necessary for them to be able to adapt to the demands made upon them. Interprofessional teams must come together to deliver care to the population.

An interprofessional team is described as follows (Taylor and Webster-Henderson 2017).

> *Team members work according to their scope of practice, share information to support each other's work and co-ordinate processes and interventions in the provision of services.*

Goodman and Clemow (2011) add that interprofessional working is when professionals collaboratively work together more effectively to improve the quality of patient care. They communicate more effectively and work in a more cohesive and productive manner.

Teams are complex and range from those that draw from a single professional group, multiprofessional teams, teams that work closely together in one place, teams that are geographically distributed, teams with constant membership and teams with constantly changing membership.

There are different types of team that collaborate to achieve what is best for the patient. They can be described as an operational team, a project team or a management team, though this is not exhaustive and the list can be extended to include self-managed teams and communities of practice.

An operational team is often seen as the 'face' of the organisation by the people who use their services.

A project team is one which comes together to develop new initiatives or undertake specific tasks. This is a particularly useful way of bringing together a variety of perspectives and ideas as well as skills and knowledge. A project team might involve a cross-section of staff carrying out tasks that are time bound. This type of team can sometimes be referred to as 'task and finish'.

A management team is likely to have more detailed objectives and development strategies; they are likely to be involved with planning operations, allocating resources and co-ordinating the work of others. Members of this team will provide day-to-day leadership and manage the boundaries between functions.

Successful teamwork has a significant and positive impact on the patient (Sun et al. 2018). This includes minimising adverse events and improving outcomes. In order to achieve the best outcome for patients and service users, it is vital that teams are effective, efficient, focused, successful, clear about aims, and can collaborate with others.

A team consists of individuals working together to accomplish a common goal or outcome. In the context of healthcare, it is about positively affecting patient outcomes by working collaboratively with other healthcare professionals. It is vital that healthcare teams understand each other's roles and responsibilities when they work together, so that they do not miss or replicate aspects of care. This also enables teams to work towards improving services.

There are many factors to consider when we look at what makes a successful team. These include but are not limited to effective communication, adhering to health and safety practices, an awareness of human and environmental factors and having a common purpose (Gluyas 2015). Measurable goals should be realistic in terms of achievement. Effective leadership is a fundamental part of an effective team. Effective leaders should set and maintain structures, manage conflict effectively, listen openly and trust and support the team members. These aspects of leadership are essential to ensure that patient safety is maintained and there are no more Francis (2013) or Berwick (2013) reports.

Highly functioning teams are known to reduce errors, increase patient safety and improve patient mortality rates, and team members have better outcomes and also have improved job satisfaction (Barr and Dowding 2022).

Teams need to function effectively to facilitate the work required of them. There are many theories of how teams form and one theory was suggested by Bruce Tuckman, a psychology professor who carried out research on team dynamics in 1965. Originally four stages were identified and in the 1970s he added a fifth. The original stages are 'forming', 'storming', 'norming' and 'performing'. The fifth 'adjourning' stage is when a team has completed the assignment or task successfully and they then disband. Members of the team then move on to new things or return to their previous position, feeling good about what has been achieved.

Another stage has been added more recently, that of 'mourning'. This is when a team has finished what they came together for and moved on. Sometimes the members of this group experience a sense of loss of the membership of the team and go through a stage of mourning (Tuckman 1965).

Teams are formed and if successful have an understanding of each member's roles and responsibilities and can therefore work together constructively. Scope of practice is key in this area – see Chapter 3 to review the importance of your scope of practice.

Another aspect of team working to consider is roles or functions. In the 1970s Dr Meredith Belbin, a management theorist, described eight roles within a team: these reflect the personality of an individual and are often assumed unconsciously. An individual can take on more than one role. This theory gives you an idea of where you fit within a team and where others fit and will help you to understand where you and others have a natural tendency to work more productively.

> *A team is not a bunch of people with job titles, but a congregation of individuals each of whom has a role which is understood by other members. Members of a team seek out certain roles & they perform more effectively in the ones that are most natural to them.*
>
> *(Dr R.M. Belbin)*

Belbin described roles and characteristics. Each role has a set of typical features, positive qualities and allowable weaknesses. For more detailed information follow the link, complete the questionnaire to see where you fit (Belbin 1993) (www.belbin.com/about/belbin-team-roles).

Reflective Activity: Being a Member of a Team

Spend some time thinking about the teams that you work in. Make a list of who is in your team. What do they do? What is their function? Who else do you come into contact with who is not in your immediate team? What are your experiences of working in different teams?

There are times when a team will develop toxic traits and become dysfunctional. In many cases the leadership style they experience will have a direct impact on the formation of the team. When a team lacks a strong leader, a more dominant member of the group can often take charge. This can lead to a lack of direction, infighting or a focus on the wrong priorities as well as poor patient care and poor adherence to procedures, guidelines and protocols.

Barriers to Team Development

There are many factors that can be a barrier to team development, including changing roles and changing settings.

Changing Roles

Changes and overlapping of roles can present challenges to teams in terms of role allocation and acknowledgement. Roles develop and evolve in response to the changing needs of service users. What once only physiotherapists did now crosses over into what an occupational therapist will do. The two professional disciplines work more closely together to provide a more comprehensive and joined-up service. One example is when they collaborate to ensure that patients have a safe and efficient discharge from acute services to the community.

Changing Settings

The nature of healthcare is changing, including increased delivery of care for people with chronic disorders in the community, increased numbers of procedures delivered in day care and community settings, the development of new teams and the increased development and modification of existing settings.

Instability of Teams

A good proportion of teams are in transition, with new starters and leavers, learners and those who work temporarily in clinical areas. In this case, development needs are variable and constantly changing, which presents the challenge

However, collaborative practice between teams is the best way to ensure that patient safety is supported and outcomes are positive. A collaborative approach serves to improve care delivery, reduce errors, increase patient safety and improve job satisfaction (Babiker et al. 2014).

Communication in Teams

Teamwork does not just happen – there needs to be an understanding of the characteristics of successful teams, knowledge of how teams function and ways to maintain effective team functioning. At the heart of this is effective open communication.

Clear communication is central to a team's ability to function and be effective. Sharing ideas and information with all members of the interdisciplinary team in a safe environment leads to positive outcomes. There should be respect for individual talents and beliefs, and an appreciation of professional contributions. This will reinforce the role each member plays in achieving the desired outcomes. Open communication in what is considered a safe environment will support ideas and opinions being shared and discussed in a professional manner. This focuses on what will be the most effective and efficient way forward for patients.

Communication strategies are important in our day-to-day work and essential in all the activities we carry out. They are linked to the standardised, practised approaches to communication that support us to work more effectively. They are there to improve communication and to make sure that information is exchanged in a professional manner.

There are many different communication tools and aids used in healthcare, but for them to be effective they need to have specific traits to avoid miscommunication. Good communication systems and strategies should be easy to understand and follow. They should offer consistency and predictability. They should feature 'redundancy' so that if the process fails in one part of the system, another part offers the opportunity for the failure to be recovered. They should incorporate forcing functions – users are steered to do the right thing in the right way. They should reduce the opportunity for 'work arounds' and reliance on memory. There are many examples of these, including one which you may be familiar with: Situation, Background, Assessment, Recommendations or Request (SBAR) – electronic forms that will not allow you to move to the next stage unless all other sections have been completed (NHS Institute for Innovation and Improvement 2023).

It is of course important that all systems used are evaluated, especially by the people who use them. Regular assessment of the suitability of equipment, processes or procedures can facilitate adjustments to ensure that what is being used is fit for purpose. Working collaboratively with manufacturers and designers can lead to more efficient products and systems that enhance patient safety and support care delivery. Being able to evaluate what you use will help you to use systems more effectively and in turn influence design and 'user friendliness' as well as practicability. This is particularly true for the NA who is based at the 'bed side' of the patient using the systems designed for them by others.

The impact on care delivery can be significant. By improving communication between all members of the care team and by communicating more effectively, the patient's experience will greatly improve. This can transform the patient journey, improve outcomes and safety and reduce errors (O'Daniel et al. 2008).

It is important to recognise the role that developing a rapport with people plays in a team's development and subsequent functioning. Rapport is the basis of meaningful, close, harmonious relationships. It supports a connection and we develop a bond; when we have a rapport with someone, it can be positive and make us feel as if we have developed a relationship with them. There are many benefits to developing a rapport with our work colleagues and team members; it fosters team cohesion, there is less conflict and a sense of empathy develops. We spend a considerable amount of time at work with our colleagues – we work together, eat together, make decisions together and share information about ourselves. Rapport can develop naturally, it can be nurtured and improved, and it can be instant or developed over time. The important point is that as members of the caring profession, we do need it and we can develop it.

Another factor that supports good communication is our emotional intelligence (EI). EI is made up of several facets, including empathy, self-awareness, motivation, self-regulation and our social skills. It is described as the 'ability of a healthcare worker to manage their emotions while interpreting and responding to those of others' (Cadman and Brewer 2001).

Emotional intelligence is not a new concept and was first described back in 1900 (Thorndike and Stein 1937). It is now recognised as being as important if not more so than our Intelligence Quotient (IQ) (Kovacs and Pléh 2023). Standardised tests are used to assess an individual's intelligence and measures their ability to apply reason – how well someone can use information and logic to answer questions. It has been identified that EI supports team working and promotes better outcomes for patients. From an organisational point of view, it encourages staff to raise issues both negative and positive, so that practices can be either promoted and shared or reviewed and changed.

There have been many technological advances in a comparatively short space of time. There is a determined move away from paper to electronically collecting and storing patient data. This includes electronic patient records, results and referrals to other services. We share information with other healthcare providers and multiagency public protection groups work together to support patients.

Police, probation service personnel, mental health staff, social services and community services work collaboratively and communicate more effectively and efficiently when they use the same electronic platform.

> ### Reflective Activity
>
> Make a list of all the ways in which you collect and store patient data.

NHS Digital (https://digital.nhs.uk) talks about data and technology that improve lives. It also looks to improve care and drive research. One of the more well-known applications is the NHS App, to get information and manage services and the 111 service for patients.

Technology has the potential to streamline services and processes, and the addition of advanced data analytical programs and the increased use of artificial intelligence will only support the development and improvement of communication systems. The use of remote consultations can address some of the issues around geographical location and those rural areas that are challenging to access or where there are fewer healthcare professionals to serve the population. The move to digital technology is about improving services and widening participation too. While this is more of a national perspective, it is important to review the way we use technology in our day-to-day interactions with patients and service users.

However, no system is flawless. There are times when technology fails and not all systems are easy to use or interact with; not all patients are entirely comfortable with the seemingly heavy reliance on technology. The data being inputted is a potential area where mistakes can occur. Ideally there should be no option for a 'work around'; however, people can be resourceful when they want to take a short cut because the perception is that 'it will be quicker than waiting for the machine'. One example is waiting for an update on services ordered for a service user or results from tests; rather than wait for a system to be updated, it could be seen as easier to telephone the department or individual for an update.

Storage of data is also a concern for patients and while we do everything possible to ensure security of data, it is sometimes the case that storage areas and systems are not secured. There are multiple reasons why this might happen but it is important to keep up to date with training on new systems, to refresh your knowledge and make sure that you are putting procedures into practice.

Critical Thinking, Problem Solving and Decision Making

Making the right decisions contributes to patient safety. We all solve problems and make decisions every day, not only in our working lives but in our day-to-day activities too. Having an opportunity to stand back and review the stages you followed will enhance your ability to continue to solve problems and give you an appreciation of the skills involved.

Critical thinking skills, critical analysis, cognitive skills and intuition are all terms used when problem solving and decision making are discussed

(Levett-Jones et al. 2010). Clinical reasoning, clinical judgement, problem solving and decision making all fit together.

Critical Thinking

Critical thinking is a skill that helps a healthcare professional to look for alternative solutions to problems by having a questioning approach. It is also necessary to communicate effectively with others in order to implement solutions for the best possible patient outcomes (Holland and Roberts 2023). You will be working in collaboration with others, potentially throughout all the stages of your career, and you will need to consider the clinical area, your own skill set and that of others, as these factors influence the options available.

Problem Solving

Problem solving is sometimes referred to as a soft skill or non-technical skill but this undermines how important this is. Patient-centred decision making is based on clinical reasoning and requires a host of skills including interpersonal, technical and cognitive (Holland and Roberts 2023).

Reflective Activity

What was your thought process when you were last faced with a problem? List the stages that you went through and the questions you asked.

The 'Clinical Reasoning Cycle' is an established tool that can support healthcare staff to make decisions. It is a process that has the following stages: consider the patient's situation; collect cues and information from various sources; process that information; identify the problem or issues; establish the goals; take actions; evaluate the outcomes; reflect on the process and identify new learning. Thompson et al. (2013) emphasise that it is important to have an understanding of the decision-making process so as to make appropriate healthcare decisions. There are several models available outlining the steps involved in the decision-making process. In 1993 Tschikota considered the various elements of decision making and identified six elements.

'*Cue*' includes all the information you can get from the patient, visually, auditory or from data collected prior to meeting the patient, including a review of written notes. With the RN, you will develop a '*hypothesis*' ('it could be...') which is based on the '*knowledge base*' that you and the RN have and involves linking the evidence or information about the patient to possibilities as to what may be creating a healthcare concern. Following the collection of data, with the RN and in collaboration with the patient, you will determine a '*nursing intervention*' and the actions that need to be taken. It is then important to '*search*' and consider anything that might be impacting on the individual. In collaboration with the RN, you will then develop an '*assumption*' based on the available information ('I think...').

The point of this cycle is that you work with the rest of the team caring for an individual and continually reflect, refine and develop your plan or intervention. There are similarities with the nursing process discussed in Chapter 3.

Any decision, whether this relates to patient care and the provision of resources or the organisation of the team, must be based on whichever option will be the most effective. It is not always the quickest or most economical option that will necessarily be the best choice. There may be choices that are more complex and expensive. You should try to avoid going for the 'quick win' merely on the basis that it is the most economical; what is important is the end-result and the long-term impact.

Choices should be made based on the most recent and viable evidence. Any decisions and judgements that you make must be supported by underpinning knowledge and evidence. There is a wealth of research and information available to support decisions and actions that are evidence based and which provide the most effective outcomes for patients.

There are an increasing number of computer-based programs that can support healthcare decision making. When considering Benner's (1982) novice to expert and competent to proficient continuum, these algorithms are helpful in supporting decision making and complementing the professional's own expertise, but they do not replace clinical judgement and clinical experience. They are there to support rather than substitute.

Evaluation is necessary and at this stage it is worth asking the question 'What worked and what hasn't worked?'. Being honest at this stage will be more valuable than trying to justify a solution that has not had the desired outcome. It is then prudent to think about recommendations moving forward. This can focus on repeating actions or what not to take forward, should the event or situation arise again.

Factors that can have a negative influence on the decision-making process include an inadequate knowledge base, inadequate skills, emotional difficulties, lack of opportunity and dependence on others. This list is not exhaustive and there are many contributing factors that should be considered.

There are also biases in our decision making that we should be aware of. These can heavily influence the decisions we make and this is why the evaluation stage is especially important (https://nshcs.hee.nhs.uk/about/equality-diversity-and-inclusion/conscious-inclusion/understanding-different-types-of-bias)

The Ishikawa Diagram, sometimes called the 'cause and effect' or fishbone diagram, is named after Kaoru Ishikawa, a Japanese industrialist who worked to revitalise the Japanese industry after the Second World War. There are five categories: What happened? Where? Who? Was there any equipment? Were there any materials used? It is useful for identifying problem areas, looking at solutions and carrying out a root cause analysis (www.youtube.com/watch?v=mLvizyDFLQ40).

Incidents and Accidents: Patient Safety Incident Response Framework (PSIRF)

Patient safety is high on the healthcare agenda, and all members of the healthcare team must be aware and develop their understanding of how multiple factors amalgamate to influence decisions and actions in healthcare that can contribute to incidents. Everyone has a duty to take actions to reduce the risk of hazards and accidents in the workplace. It is also important to know what individual responsibilities are and the role everyone plays in the prevention of incidents. Behind the policies and procedures that guide and inform practice is a raft of legislation and guidelines. These translate into procedures, policies and protocols to promote safe working practices for the sake of your patients, visitors and other staff members.

Safety is not a standalone discipline and health and safety are integrated into all aspects of care. There are multiple agencies that have an influence on safety, including the National Patient Safety Agency (NHS Improvement) and the MHRA (Medicines and Healthcare Products Regulatory Agency). The professional bodies also have a significant role to play, including the Nursing and Midwifery Council (NMC), the General Medical Council (GMC) and the Health and Care Professionals Council (HCPC). Professional standards including the NMC Code (2018) state our duty to safeguard, and be accountable for our own actions, omissions and limitations.

In 1709, Alexander Pope coined the phrase 'To err is human ...' (Croskerry 2010) and Sir Liam Donaldson (2002) talked about organisations with a memory in respect of incidents and patient safety and how the highly complex and technical field of medicine must be aware of the importance of systems failure in the areas of accidents.

Errors fall into two categories: human or technical. Most incidents are due to a series of failings. Reason's Swiss cheese model (1997), explains that errors often occur as a result of failings in systems and which he called 'latent errors'. The model is based on an understanding that every step in a process or layer of a system has a weakness that can potentially lead to failure. Reason likened processes or systems to slices of Swiss cheese laid side by side. The holes in the Swiss cheese represent potential weaknesses at each particular stage or layer. Some of these holes are considered 'active' – an individual making an error – and others are considered 'latent'. These weaknesses are inherent to the system and may include poor organisational design or weak management systems. According to this model, a series of barriers are in place to prevent hazards from causing harm to humans. The presence of the holes in one slice of cheese does not normally lead to a poor outcome, but if by chance all the holes are aligned, the hazard reaches the patient and causes harm.

If one of the holes is penetrated, a failure will occur at that point. The chances are that the layer behind will block any further failure. Each slice of 'cheese' acts as a 'defence' against further failure and represents an opportunity to stop or avoid an error. But if the holes in each layer come into alignment, the potential for failure at each and every stage becomes real.

The aim of risk management is to reduce harm to patients and ensure their safety. While we cannot remove all risk, we can use tools and assessments to guide actions in reducing the risks. These include the Safer Surgery checklist (WHO 2008), SBAR and other risk assessments to indicate appropriate actions to take to reduce the potential for error (NHS Institute for Innovation and Improvement 2023). Some of these systems serve to negate the error from both technical and human perspectives.

Human factors are sometimes called ergonomics. This includes equipment, workspaces, workplace practices, organisational structure, safety procedures and training. Human factors is a discipline in itself and not a new topic. 'Human factors refer to environmental, organisational and job factors, and human and individual characteristics, which influence behaviour at work in a way which can affect health and safety' (HSE 2022). Human factors are organisational, individual, environmental and job characteristics that influence behaviour in ways that can impact safety (https://youtu.be/aGZz3w5Hy8Y).

Studying human factors and understanding the role they play in patient safety can reduce the number of incidents experienced every year. However, deviations do occur. There may be system flaws, poor understanding, insufficient peer control of reckless or overconfident individuals, boundaries of safe practice being breached and a lack of engagement with human factors, including a lack of situational awareness, flawed decision making, inexperience, dysfunctional team working, poor problem solving, poor communication and a lack of effective leadership.

Following protocols, policies or care bundles creates a systems approach that can reduce the incidence of accidents. There is also 'foresight training' which places more of a focus on the individual. Human factors training allows for the development of skills so that practitioners can be proactive in promoting patient safety and reducing incidents. Foresight training was developed to improve awareness of the factors that might cause harm to a patient. It is also about empowering staff to intervene to prevent patients from suffering harm. It can increase local learning by sharing experiences and improving understanding of risk-prone and near-miss situations. It helps nurses, nursing associates and midwives to adopt a more proactive approach to managing complex dynamic healthcare systems.

Foresight is the ability to:

- recognise potential risks to patient safety in the healthcare system
- identify and respond to initial indications that a patient safety incident could take place
- intervene and recover to prevent a patient safety incident.

Another factor around safety is staff numbers and an understanding of safe staffing is important. It is more than just numbers of staff – it is about having the right staff with the right skills in the right place at the right time to meet the needs of the patient population being cared for. It should not be viewed as a stand-alone area but as an integral part of patient and staff safety. NICE guidelines and NHS Improvement provide definitions and detail to allow staff to look at their areas from a wider perspective. Follow this link for more information: www.england.nhs.uk/nursingmidwifery/safer-staffing-nursing-and-midwifery

Another element of human factors is having a safety culture at work. Amy Edmondson's pioneering work into psychological safety in the workplace describes it as 'a belief that one will not be punished, blamed or humiliated for speaking up with ideas, questions, concerns or mistakes'. Over the last 20 years, Edmondson has investigated a wide range of organisations to identify why they are psychologically safe learning cultures. Her work commenced in healthcare in America where she was employed as part of a research project looking into medication errors and how they could be reduced (Edmondson 2018). Edmondson found that those areas with a high reporting rate of incidents were more open to questions and challenge of themselves and their colleagues than those with a low reporting rate. Team members should feel included, safe to learn, safe to contribute, safe to challenge – all of this is part of creating a positive culture.

Psychological safety is essential for creating effective leadership and learning cultures. It influences proactive behaviours (asking questions, reporting errors, open communication) and is associated with strong interpersonal relationships which in turn create effective cultures that include collaboration, trust and innovation.

NHS England (2023) identifies that innovation is critical to enabling the NHS to achieve the ambitions set out in the Mandate, to ramp up the pace and scale of change, and deliver better outcomes for patients across all five domains of the NHS Outcomes Framework. The NHS is a major investor and wealth creator in the UK, and in science, technology and engineering in particular. It is possible that with change and improvement, errors can be reduced, patient safety can be increased and there will be improved job satisfaction.

Patient safety is about maximising the things that go right and minimising the things that go wrong. It is integral to the NHS's definition of quality in healthcare, alongside effectiveness and patient experience. Improvements need to be worked on from a collaborative point of view. The NHS Accelerated Access Collaborative stated: 'We're bringing together industry, government, regulators, patients and the NHS to remove barriers and accelerate the introduction of ground-breaking new treatments and diagnostics which can transform care'. Innovation can increase patient safety and lead to improved services. When we consider improvement, it is pertinent to look at national recommendations as well as what can be improved for the local population.

- How do we know what needs to be improved? What mechanisms are in place to inform improvement initiatives and change?
- The NHS Long Term Plan: talks about improving services and is very specific about the areas where improvement needs to take plaace.
- The NHS Outcomes Framework talks about 'treating and caring for people in a safe environment and protecting them from avoidable harm' (domain 5).

Culture

Culture is often described as the characteristics and knowledge of a particular group of people. This usually includes language, religion, cuisine, social habits, music, arts, outlook, attitudes, values, moral goals and customs. Sometimes it is stated as 'the way we do things around here'.

It is suggested that shared values, beliefs and norms influence the way employees think, feel and act towards others inside and outside the organisation.

Some elements of an organisation that make up the culture include stories, rituals and routines, symbols, organisational structure, control systems and power structures. All of these elements link to the organisation's values. Unfortunately, there have been instances where the cultures within particular organisations have been harmful and toxic. The Francis report and others which followed have laid bare the impact a toxic culture has had on patient care and safety.

To ensure that organisational cultures develop in a more productive and positive manner, the vision of the organisation needs to be communicated effectively to all. Not only that, but it is essential that all members understand what the vision is and their role in achieving it. The vision also needs to be revisited to ensure that it remains relevant to the needs of service users or patients. Moving towards a 'no blame' culture will have a positive influence on how organisations develop, grow and increase patient safety.

By acknowledging and owning problems, it becomes possible to address the issues and take the right actions. Asking 'why' this happened allows us to address issues and make the changes necessary to change or improve the delivery of care.

The relatively new Patient Safety Incident Response Framework (PSIRF), while not solely about culture, does link to the issue of patient safety and how organisations can change the way they look at issues and take a different approach to learning and improvement. When mistakes are reframed as learning opportunities, it moves away from a blame culture and fosters a more open culture and in turn resilient workforce (www.england.nhs.uk/patient-safety/patient-safety-insight/incident-response-framework).

When considering culture, it is also necessary to be aware of potential conflict; conflict is a fact of life and can arise anywhere. Conflict can be described as a struggle between people which may be physical or between conflicting ideas. Conflict can arise because there are needs, values or ideas that are seen to be different, and there is no means to reconcile the dispute.

There are several ways to resolve conflict and an individual may have a leaning towards one of the following styles.

- *Avoiding*: 'Maybe the problem will go away.'
- *Accommodating*: 'Let's do it your way.' Sometimes described as co-operative but unassertive. This style tends to be self-sacrificing to meet the other's goals; it is appropriate especially if the other individual is right.
- *Compromising*: 'Let's split the difference.' Assertive and co-operative. This allows both parties to feel they have made sacrifices for agreement. A lose–lose strategy.
- *Collaborating*: 'Let's co-operate to reach a win–win solution that benefits both of us.' This is assertive and co-operative. It allows problems to be identified and alternatives to be explored until difficulties are resolved. Win–win strategy.
- *Competing*: assertive and unco-operative. This power-orientated style is appropriate if the situation needs a quick or unpopular decision. However, if used too often, colleagues become afraid of admitting to making mistakes. Win–lose strategy.

Nursing associates need to have an awareness of conflict and to know how people act when they are exposed to conflict. You may have an opportunity to resolve conflict between staff and potentially between patients, clients or service users.

Leadership, Psychological Safety, Learning Environments, Change and Improvements

Good leadership can result in patients being more satisfied, reduced mortality rates, patient safety improves and staff have better health and wellbeing. There is lower absenteeism and as a consequence individual Trusts have better financial performance (NHS Healthcare Leadership model – www.leadershipacademy. nhs.uk/healthcare-leadership-model).

A good leader should be able to think critically, solve problems, respect people, communicate skilfully, set goals, share visions and develop themselves and others (Whitehead et al. 2019). A good leader is said to have the following characteristics: confidence, be able to advocate, be assertive, have empathy, be supportive, be focused, be fair, be knowledgeable, be able to analyse and have integrity. They must also recognise the skills that others have and know when to allow others to lead in any given situation. Leadership is not solely dependent upon an individual's seniority.

There has been a shift in the focus of leaders, away from targets and more towards consideration for staff members.

There are many theories and styles of leadership. One is the transformational leader which is based around the leader being proactive. This leadership style works to change the organisational culture by implementing new ideas and this leader can motivate and empower staff to achieve objectives by appealing to higher ideals and values. They also motivate by appealing to the interest of others; these leaders will support change in the way people see things or situations and challenge 'the way things are' or the existing structure. They inspire and encourage creativity among staff and have the ability to share power and offer encouragement. They act as a role model and can clearly communicate and share a vision and goals, building trust within the team. The decision-making process and planning are shared. This style of leadership creates more positive outcomes for teams and interactions between members.

Leadership is integral to establishing effective and efficient teamwork; a leader needs followers and the followers need to understand what the leader is in pursuit of. This links to what you have learnt in this chapter about communication, teamwork and culture. Being able to communicate a clear vision, establish shared values and goals and an understanding of the desired outcome all contribute to a fully functioning team that promotes patient safety, learning and cohesion. This also supports innovation, improvement and promotes a psychologically safe environment where learning can take place and the team can grow and develop.

A good leader creates an environment where staff are able to speak up and challenge, to support safety and good practice alongside improvements in care delivery.

There are other leadership styles which may be relevant in specific situations.

Autocratic

This is a very 'top-down' approach, which tends to be controlling. This may be necessary in emergency situations where leadership by an experienced member of the team is needed.

Democratic

This type of leader makes decisions by consulting their team while still maintaining control of the group. A good democratic leader encourages participation from all staff and motivates the team by empowering them to direct themselves. The downside is that this process can be time-consuming and may not be appropriate in some clinical situations.

Laissez Faire

The leader has minimal influence and sometimes has a very 'hands-off' approach. They tend to be non-directive or inactive. While this may work with a well-established highly motivated team and will support autonomy, it can lead to a lack of direction and the team can quickly become non-productive. There is little control over the team, leaving them to sort out their roles and responsibilities which can leave them floundering with little direction or motivation. It can lead to frustration amongst team members, particularly if there is a clash between values and work ethic. This approach can be effective when leading a team of highly motivated or skilled workers. Groups of fully autonomous and independent care workers can feel empowered to make decisions. This style works best when people are capable and motivated and there is no requirement for central co-ordination.

Reflective Activity

Perhaps there are changes that you would like to see in your own clinical area. Or perhaps you have been involved in changes to practice yourself. Think about this and see if you can answer the following questions.

- How did it come about?
- What was the purpose of the change?
- How did it make you feel?
- What were/are the benefits of the change?
- What was it?
- What were the barriers/resistance to the change?
- Did it go well?
- What did you do?
- How did the change take place?

How do we achieve change and improvement? Everyone has a role to play in achieving the desired results. It is important to examine the importance of working with others in teams to deliver and improve services. What is known is that changes in the culture of the NHS and social care are required if improvements to care are to be meaningful and lasting.

Change does need to be managed and there are several theories of change that can be utilised. One example is Lewin's change model which is a straightforward three-stage model (Hussain et al. 2018). The three stages can be used effectively to ensure that lasting changes are brought about that will enhance patient care, support staff and reflect innovation and improvement as well as reducing patient safety incidents.

- *Stage 1 – unfreeze*: this is preparing the team/area for the change, ensuring that team members understand the need for the change. Good communication is key. This is usually the most stressful time for both the team and the change agent as values, beliefs, attitudes and behaviours may be challenged.
- *Stage 2 – change*: in order for this stage to work and for people to contribute, they need to understand how it will benefit them. They also need to know what is coming, any rumours must be dispelled.
- *Stage 3 – refreeze*: the change now needs to be maintained. Evaluate progress and establish feedback systems, ensuring everyone is informed and supported.

However, change can be met with resistance and according to Kotter and Schlesinger (1989), there are four common reasons for this: not wanting to give up something of personal value; a misunderstanding about the importance of the change; a belief that the change will not benefit the organisation; or a low tolerance for change. There are, of course, other possibilities which can include past experience or the change being perceived as a threat to someone's autonomy or power.

Stability, order and support are important as any change can threaten these. A change may signal the need to learn new skills or procedures.

Improving care delivery and services is part of the government's national agenda. All healthcare professionals have a role to play. Having an understanding of why change is needed will support the NA and other members of the interdisciplinary team to implement and manage change.

Chapter Summary

This chapter has explored the nature of teams and the importance of working collaboratively to ensure that patients remain at the heart of what healthcare professionals do. You have had the opportunity to reflect on the importance of effective teams in ensuring patient safety and the safety of those working within the healthcare team. The NA is ideally placed to deliver, monitor and contribute to patient safety. The chapter explored leadership styles and how these contribute to different aspects of patient safety and change within the workplace. It also considered the importance of effective change and how the NA can be involved in supporting change within the team.

References

Babiker, A., El Husseini, M., Al Nemri, A. et al. (2014). Health care professional development: working as a team to improve patient care. *Sudan Journal of Paediatrics* 14 (2): 9–16.

Barr, J. and Dowding, L. (2022). *Leadership in Health Care*, 5e. London: Sage.

Belbin, R.M. (1993). *Team Roles at Work*. Oxford: Butterworth-Heinemann.

Benner, P. (1982). From novice to expert. *American Journal of Nursing* 82 (3): 402–407.

Berwick, D. (2013). *A Promise to Learn – A Commitment to Act. Improving the Safety of Patients in England*. London: National Advisory Group on the Safety of Patients in England.

Cadman, C. and Brewer, J. (2001). Emotional intelligence: a vital prerequisite for recruitment in nursing. *Journal of Nursing Management* 9: 321–324.

Croskerry P. (2010). To err is human–and let's not forget it. *CMAJ* 182(5): 524. doi: 10.1503/cmaj.100270.

Donaldson, L. (2002). An organisation with a memory. *Clinical Medicine* 2 (5): 452–457.

Edmondson, A.C. (2018). *The Fearless Organization: Creating Psychological Safety in the Workplace for Learning, Innovation, and Growth*. Hoboken: John Wiley & Sons.

Francis, R. (2013). *Report of the Mid Staffordshire NHS Foundation Trust Public Inquiry: Executive Summary (HC 947)*. London: Stationery Office.

Gluyas, H. (2015). Effective communication and teamwork promotes patient safety. *Nursing Standard* 29: 50–57.

Goodman, B. and Clemow, R. (2011). *Nursing and Collaborative Practice*, 2e. Exeter: Learning Matters.

Health and Safety Executive (HSE) (2022). Human factors and ergonomics. www.hse.gov.uk/humanfactors/

Holland, K. and Roberts, D. (2023). *Decision-making in Nursing Practice*. London:: Sage.

Hussain, S.T., Lei, S., Akram, T. et al. (2018). Kurt Lewin's change model: a critical review of the role of leadership and employee involvement in organizational change. *Journal of Innovation and Knowledge* 3 (3): 123–127.

Kotter, J.P. and Schlesinger, L.A. (1989). Choosing strategies for change. In: *Readings in Strategic Management* (ed. D. Asch and C. Bowman). London: Palgrave.

Kovacs, K. and Pléh, C. (2023). William Stern: the relevance of his program of 'differential psychology' for contemporary intelligence measurement and research. *Journal of Intelligence* 11 (3): 41.

Levett-Jones, T., Hoffman, K., Dempsey, J. et al. (2010). The 'five rights' of clinical reasoning: an educational model to enhance nursing students' ability to identify and manage clinically 'at risk' patients. *Nurse Education Today* 30 (6): 515–520.

NHS Institute for Innovation and Improvement (2023). Safer Care. SBAR: Situation, Background, Assessment, Recommendations. Implementation and Training Guide. www.england.nhs.uk/improvement-hub/wp-content/uploads/sites/44/2017/11/SBAR-Implementation-and-Training-Guide.pdf

Nursing and Midwifery Council (NMC) (2018). *The Code: Professional Standards of Practice and Behaviour for Nurses, Midwives and Nursing Associates*. London: Nursing and Midwifery Council.

O'Daniel, M., Rosenstein, A.H., and Hughes, R. (ed.) (2008). Professional communication and team collaboration. In: *Patient Safety and Quality: An Evidence-Based Handbook for Nurses*. Rockville: Agency for Healthcare Research and Quality.

Reason, J.T. (1997). *Managing the Risks of Organisational Accidents.* Aldershot: Ashgate.

Sun, R., Marshall, D.C., Sykes, M.C., and Maruthappu, J.S. (2018). The impact of improving teamwork on patient outcomes in surgery: a systematic review. *International Journal of Surgery* 53: 171–177.

Taylor, R. and Webster-Henderson, B. (2017). *The Essentials of Nursing Leadership.* London: Sage.

Thompson, C., Aitken, L., Doran, D., and Dowding, D. (2013). An agenda for clinical decision making and judgement in nursing research and education. *International Journal of Nursing Studies* 50 (12): 1720–1726.

Thorndike, R.L. and Stein, S. (1937). An evaluation of the attempts to measure social intelligence. *Psychological Bulletin* 34: 275–285.

Tuckman, B. (1965). Developmental sequence in small groups. *Psychological Bulletin* 63: 384–399.

Walsh, N. and de Sarandy, S. (2023). The practice of collaborative leadership: across health and care services. www.kingsfund.org.uk/insight-and-analysis/reports/practice-collaborative-leadership

Whitehead, D., Weiss, S., and Tappen, K. (2019). *Essentials of Nursing Leadership and Management*, 7e. Philadelphia: F.A. Davis.

World Health Organization (WHO) (2008). Safe Surgery: Tool and Resources. Surgical Safety Checklist. www.who.int/teams/integrated-health-services/patient-safety/research/safe-surgery/tool-and-resources

Further Reading

Bibi, S., Comley, E., and Forman, J. (2023). *Team Working and Professional Practice for Nursing Associates.* London: Sage.

Cowls, H., Tobin, S., and Cusack, N. (2024). *Understanding Leadership for Nursing Associates.* London: Sage.

Eliis, P. (2022). *Leadership, Management and Team Working*, 4e. London: Sage.

Ellis, P. (2023). *Evidence-Based Practice in Nursing*, 5e. London: Sage/Learning Matters.

Fisher, M. and Scott, M. (2013). *Patient Safety and Managing Risk in Nursing.* London: Sage/Learning Matters.

Gopee, N. and Galloway, J. (2017). *Leadership and Management in Healthcare*, 3e. London: Sage.

Huber, D. (2018). *Leadership and Nursing Care Management*, 6e. London: Saunders.

Janes, G. and Delves-Yates, C. (ed.) (2023). *Quality Improvement in Nursing.* London: Sage/Learning Matters.

Kelly, P. and Tazbir, J. (ed.) (2021). *Nursing Leadership and Management*, 4e. Oxford: Willey-Blackwell.

Metcalf-Alban, J. (2018). Engaging leadership – a better approach to leading a team? *Nursing Times* 114 (6): 21–24.

Owens, M., Adams, J., Rogers, P. et al. (2024). *Understanding Evidence-Based Practice.* London: Sage.

Peate, I. (2019). *Learning to Care: The Nursing Associate.* Edinburgh: Elsevier.

Peate, I. (2020). *Assessment and Care Planning for Nurses.* Oxford: Wiley Blackwell.

Peate, I. (2021). *The Nursing Associate at a Glance.* Oxford: Wiley Blackwell.

Rixon, J. (2023). The leadership role and development for the registered nursing associate. *British Journal of Nursing* 32 (10,): 484–485.

Yoder-Wise, P. (ed.) (2019). *Leading and Managing in Nursing,*, 7e. St Louis: Mosby Elsevier.

8 Nursing Associates and the Importance of Being Curious

Rose Webster

University Hospitals of Leicester NHS Trust, Leicester, UK

Introduction

One of the outcomes of the journey to becoming a nursing associate (NA) is developing an understanding of the decisions made about care. The theoretical and practical components of your Foundation degree will have exposed you to some of the latest knowledge and thinking in relation to care delivery. As a graduate, you will have experience of finding answers to the Who? What? Where? When? Why? and How? questions which form the basis of developing knowledge. You will have been encouraged to be curious and to ask questions. Think back to your course work where you used evidence from a range of sources to inform your thinking and started to develop a theoretical basis for your role. Working as a learner across all four fields of practice will have provided you with opportunities to link this theory to practice. You may have observed inconsistencies in care delivery and mismatches between what you learned and what you experienced in practice. You may have started to think critically about what makes care safe and effective in a range of different care settings.

The challenge as a (registered) NA is to continue to be curious and questioning. It is expected that you will use knowledge and skills that are clinically credible and to do this you will need up-to-date evidence to inform the care that you give. This is clearly articulated in the Nursing and Midwifery Council Standards of Proficiency for the Registered NA role (NMC 2018a).

Aims of This Chapter

- To give you the knowledge and skills to appreciate the sources of evidence that have the potential to influence care provided in your clinical working environment and the wider health and care landscape.

The Nursing Associate: Stepping into Practice, First Edition. Edited by Annabel Coulson.
© 2025 John Wiley & Sons Ltd. Published 2025 by John Wiley & Sons Ltd.

- To support you in appreciating the part you can play in evidence-based practice through being curious, asking questions and understanding how to find the best evidence to support what you and others do.
- To look at the significance of applying evidence-based practice in improving the quality of care delivery. To explore the key challenges in making this happen.

Related NMC Standards

Platform 1: (Nursing Associates Registered) ... act professionally at all times and use their knowledge and experience to make evidence-based decisions and solve problems.

Reflective Activity

Reflecting on yourself, either as a student or registrant:

- As a NA, to what extent do you use evidence to inform your practice or solve problems?
- Has the theoretical knowledge you gained as a student led you to change your practice? If so, was this change easy to make?
- Have you observed care delivered in a new way and you do not fully understand why?
- Have you voiced questions about the rationale for an aspect of care to those you work with? Have you been given clear answers?
- How do you feel about your ability to challenge practice that you believe to be potentially inappropriate, ineffective or unsafe?

Your answers to these questions will tell you something about the reality of using evidence in your day-to-day clinical practice and will perhaps inform how you use this chapter.

Evidence-based practice is relevant to your role in several ways. As a student NA, you will have focused on gaining knowledge and understanding of care that is particularly relevant to your role. When registered, you will have a role as a practice supervisor, and you will be asked questions by a range of learners working alongside you. NAs work in teams and appreciating the rationale behind care given by other healthcare professionals can support a cohesive approach to care and effective team working. Understanding the evidence behind clinical care will help you provide answers to service user questions and support them in making informed decisions. You are likely to work with individuals with a wide range of care needs and you will not remember all the knowledge relevant to their care. Knowing where to look for the best evidence and then appreciating how to use it to inform practice is an important part of your role.

The chapter starts by giving the background to evidence-based practice and highlighting its key components. It builds on this to encourage you to ask questions about the care that you give; to think about the best evidence to help answer these questions and where to find it. The factors that influence whether a particular individual at a particular time receives optimum evidence-based care are complex. This chapter discusses some of the factors that influence the use of evidence in practice, including the role of clinical decision making.

Evidence-based practice is not an isolated topic and other themes within this book have a clear evidence base, meaning that there will be links to other chapters. The content has been informed by the experience of delivering an evidence-based practice module to student NAs and the questions and examples from practice are theirs. I am grateful to the learners for sharing their experiences with me.

What Is Evidence-based Practice?

When thinking about a concept like evidence-based practice, it is useful to consider its meaning and to understand how it developed, so that your role in using evidence in practice can be seen in context.

The aim of evidence-based practice is to support clinical decision making and the evaluation of services. This is to maximise the appropriate use of resources and promote effective and safe care delivery and needs to be considered within the context of rising public expectations of healthcare and finite resources.

Historical reviews of evidence-based practice highlight the influence of the Canadian physician Gordon Guyatt who first used the term 'evidence-based medicine' in a paper that he wrote in 1991 (Guyatt 1991). Evidence-based medicine was defined in 1996 as 'the conscientious, explicit and judicious use of current best evidence in making decisions about the care of individual patients' (Sackett et al. 1996, p.72). This highlights the significance of the critical thinking behind any decision to use (or not use) evidence and the importance of transparency in the decision-making process. It also emphasises the fact that each patient or service user needs to be considered as an individual. The concept of evidence-based practice evolved with the definition provided by the British public health physician Muir Gray in 1997, who further emphasised the significance of patient involvement in informing the decision-making process.

> *Evidence based practice is an approach to decision making in which the clinician uses the best evidence available, in consultation with the patient, to decide upon the option which suits the patient best.*
> (Muir Gray 1997, p.3).

Historical Context of Evidence-based Practice

Those involved in caring for others have always hoped they were providing the best care in the circumstances they were in. However, in the last 30 years there has been a shift from care decisions based on the experience of individual clinicians and local custom, towards a culture that expects health-care to be informed by evidence that has been shown to be effective, particularly when compared to other interventions. There is a growing emphasis on making improvements in care quality and safety, while also reducing costs and variations in healthcare outcomes. These trends have been influenced by political, economic, education and public health agendas. They have been supported by developments in digital technology that have provided a route for the dissemination and critical review of clinical practice throughout the healthcare community.

Evidence-based Nursing Practice

The term 'evidence-based nursing practice' (EBNP) is sometimes applied to the use of evidence that informs nursing care. Evidence-informed practice (EIP) is an evolving concept seen as an alternative to EBP (WHO 2022). The Royal College of Nursing (RCN) highlights the fact that nursing is a safety-critical profession, with the application of evidence-based knowledge, professional and clinical judgement playing a significant part in the provision of high-quality person-centred care (RCN 2023).

A questioning approach to nursing care is not new. Florence Nightingale is remembered for her pioneering analytical approach to her work in the 1850s during the Crimean War. She did this through systematic data collection which she used as evidence to inform changes in practice, particularly around hygiene and wound care. Key to her success in this was her ability to communicate her findings effectively to those with the authority, resources and motivation to bring about change – an early example of successfully navigating the theory–practice gap.

Developments in nurse education in the 1970s and 1980s established nursing as an applied science. The first English university departments of nursing were founded in the early 1970s and like other practice professions, nursing aimed to have a knowledge base founded on theoretical concepts. The evidence for nursing practice has developed from both art and science disciplines (e.g. psychology, sociology and biology). The requirement from 2013 for all RNs to be graduates supported further academic growth in nursing, with more opportunity for postgraduate study. As an NA, you will be eligible for further graduate-level study. As well as exposing you to more evidence to support your practice, this may give you the opportunity to carry out literature reviews and possibly small-scale research studies, service improvement projects or audit as part of your studies. While it is not expected that all those in nursing roles will carry out research themselves, there is an expectation that all will have the understanding to be able to use best evidence to inform their practice (NMC 2018b). There is increased support for nurses to remain in clinical roles while being involved in research. This includes opportunities for part-time doctoral study and established academic career pathways (Avery et al. 2021).

Key Moments in the Development of Evidence-based Practice in Nursing

- **1800s:** Florence Nightingale identified a systematic approach that sought to improve the quality of healthcare.
- **1944**: The UK Medical Research Council (MRC) published a trial of patulin for the common cold. This was the first double-blind controlled trial.
- **1947:** The first international guidance on the ethics of medical research involving subjects – the Nuremberg Code – was formulated.
- **Early 1970s:** Cochrane – basing decisions on evidence; start of systematic reviews to find the best evidence for practice.
- **1971:** The first nursing research unit in the UK at the University of Edinburgh.
- **1972:** The Briggs Committee suggests a move to degree preparation of nurses – practice to be based on research (HMSO 1972).
- **1970s:** Royal College of Nursing (RCN) study of nursing care series, e.g. Stockwell (1972) The unpopular patient; Haywood (1975) Information as a prescription against pain.
- **1970s and 1980s:** Advanced clinical practice roles in nursing started to be developed with the introduction of specialist roles for nurses; these tended to have a research/EBP component.
- **1984:** First edition of *The Royal Marsden Manual of Clinical Nursing Procedures* published.
- **1996:** Sackett and colleagues defined evidence-based medicine as a concept (Sackett et al. 1996).
- **1996:** The RCN defined EBNP as 'Doing the right thing in the right way for the right patient at the right time' (RCN 1996).
- **1999:** The first NICE guidelines developed; first nurse consultants in the UK – part of their remit was research and service evaluation.
- **2001:** A range of national service frameworks developed by the Department of Health – included recognition (evidence) and support for specialist nursing roles within specific services.
- **2012–13:** All nursing courses in the UK become degree level – linked to university academic departments.
- **2015:** Shape of Caring Review; focus on supporting nursing research (Health Education England 2015).
- **2018:** Council of Deans launch clinical academic research careers for nursing, midwifery and allied health.
- **2018:** NMC Standards of Proficiency for NAs; stipulate that NAs will provide evidence-based care (NMC 2018a).
- **2018:** The National Institute for Health Care Research (NIHR) academy launched; now called the National Institute for Health and Care Research.
- **2019:** NHS Long Term Plan; funding for evidence-based health promotion, including smoking cessation, obesity reduction and diabetes (NHS England 2019).

- **2020:** The WHO introduces evidence-informed practice into its competency framework.
- **2020:** NHS England and NHS Improvement: Leading the acceleration of evidence into practice: a guide for executive nurses. Written to support leaders in putting a greater focus on research and evidence in practice. (NHS England and NHS Improvement 2020).
- **2021:** Making research matter: Chief Nursing Officer for England's strategic plan for research (NHS England 2021).
- **2021:** The Future of Clinical Research Delivery 2022–2025 published by the UK Government and devolved administrations Department of Health and Social Care, The Executive Office (Northern Ireland), The Scottish Government and Welsh Government (2021).
- **2024–2027:** RCN Research Strategy, to promote 'the voice of nursing' within research; to develop high-quality evidence and support research education, careers and leadership for nurses (RCN 2024).

Using Evidence in Practice

There are various ways in which you may engage with evidence-based practice as a NA. These include the following.

Being Aware of the Evidence Underpinning your Practice

As an accountable practitioner, you need to be able to justify decisions about the care you give and the advice and information you provide. This involves using evidence-based recommendations to inform care. This evidence might be found in sources such as policies or guidelines, reports or systematic reviews of the literature.

Finding Evidence to Support your Practice

If you are not sure about why you are doing something, particularly if you cannot find any evidence in the policies or guidelines that you use, you will start to have questions about your practice (Who? What? Where? When? Why? How?). Evidence needs to build on what is already known and a starting point is to look at what information is already available and how the question has been answered by others. This evidence is likely to come from published evidence or expert opinion from those working in similar circumstances.

Evaluating the Available Evidence

Any evidence that you do find should be looked at critically to consider if it is current, credible and applicable to your particular situation and the question you are asking, i.e. is it the 'best' evidence for you to use?

Finding New Evidence

If the available evidence does not fully address your question, there is justification for looking for new evidence. Finding the answer to a particular question will provide a new knowledge base for a specific clinical scenario.

Translating Evidence into Practice

When there is good-quality evidence to inform practice, the next step is to apply this knowledge at a local level to inform decisions about care. This may require challenging current care practices and behaviours.

Monitoring Evidence-based Practice

Once the best way of doing things has been identified and introduced into care delivery, it is good practice to monitor to see if this practice is beneficial for patient care and if it continues over time. This is achieved through service evaluation projects and audit.

What Is the Evidence Base for Practice?

It is generally agreed that evidence for care comes from a combination of sources.

- Evidence from a systematic (organised and structured) approach which involves asking clear questions and finding focused answers. This is most often carried out through a rigorous and well-organised research process.
- Evidence from those working in practice, using clinical expertise built up over time and experience in a particular clinical field.
- Evidence from patient or service user experience, preference and values formed through personal lived experience of health or illness and care delivery.

These factors are sometimes referred to, and represented by, the three legs of a stool which suggests that they are of equal importance (to give balance). However, evidence from the three sources may be of variable quality and can be seen as unequal in value. All sources of evidence have their strengths and weaknesses and the challenge is to use the most appropriate evidence in any given situation. The individual's healthcare needs and circumstances, as well as the culture of the care setting, are significant considerations in this.

One of the considerations in deciding the best evidence to use is being clear about the specific question being asked and why you are asking it.

Reflective Activity

Think about something that you do every day in practice.

- Do you have questions about the Who? What? Where? When? Why? and How? in relation to this?
- Write down a question that you have about this particular area of practice.

Students have asked the following questions about their practice which will be used to give context throughout this chapter.

- Do nurses working in mental health inpatient settings perform hand hygiene as effectively as nurses in medical ward environments?
- How often should I be repositioning patients at risk of pressure ulcers on my frail elderly ward? I have seen different timings in different clinical areas.
- Why does my community alternative placement use a different wound dressing to the one that I use in my base surgical ward?
- Why are parents and carers not bringing their children to our clinic for the MMR vaccination?

Finding the Evidence for Practice

Clinical Policies and Guidelines as a Source of Evidence for Practice

Clinical policies and guidelines aim to be a source of comprehensive, systematically developed evidence-based recommendations for clinical practice. They are intended to support consistent decision making across a range of topics with recommendations based on credible evidence from systematic research, the views of clinical experts and patient and public opinion. Clinical policies tend to be written for specific service users within local settings, whereas clinical guidelines are more broadly focused and therefore less prescriptive in their recommendations. The implementation of guidelines in clinical practice is known to be variable (Cassidy et al. 2021) and it is acknowledged that teamwork and engagement between colleagues influence this in practice (Kitson et al. 2021).

The ultimate decision about what to do in practice needs to be made in the light of individual service users' circumstances and the care options available. While professional bodies do develop clinical guidelines (for example, the European Society of Cardiology (ESC) guidelines for acute coronary syndrome (ESC 2023) and the National Clinical Guideline for Stroke for the UK and Ireland (Intercollegiate Stroke Working Party 2023)), by far the most significant provider of clinical guidelines in the UK is the National Institute for Health and Care Excellence (NICE).

NICE is an independent body responsible for providing evidence-based clinical guidelines that focus on decision making and effective use of resources in the treatment and care of people with specific diseases and conditions within the NHS in England. There are over 350 clinical guidelines available. In addition to the recommendations, NICE guidelines also summarise the evidence behind the recommendations and explain how the recommendations were derived from this evidence. There is a manual outlining the well-established process of NICE guideline development (NICE 2014).

NICE actively searches for new evidence and monitors key events (such as ongoing research studies) that are judged relevant to the guideline. Developments in digital technology have made it possible to provide links to new evidence prior to updating the guidelines in full.

It is likely that clinical guidelines will not yet include specific recommendations for the NA role (although local clinical policies might). Therefore, any recommendations need to be considered in relation to your scope of practice before you start to incorporate them into your care.

It may be that you can be involved in clinical policy or guideline development as part of your role, particularly if you develop an interest in a particular area of care, for example as a link nurse. This is a good opportunity to work with others and experience the realities of project management in practice. Finding out about the policies or guidelines used in similar clinical areas is a good start. There is likely to be an established process to follow that considers the relevant evidence and input from clinical experts, service users and those likely to use the document. You will need to consider finance and the use of resources, as well as any training and development needed to support the recommended practice.

There are several factors to consider when thinking about policy and guideline development or reviewing an existing document. The list below is based on the domains of the Agree Reporting Checklist (Brouwers et al. 2016).

Domain 1: Scope and Purpose of the Document

- Are the overall objective(s) of the guideline(s) specifically described?
- Has the health question(s) covered by the guideline been specifically described?
- Is the population (patients, public, etc.) to whom the guideline is meant to apply specifically described, e.g., age, clinical condition, place of care?

Domain 2: Stakeholder Involvement

- Does the guideline development group include individuals from all relevant professional groups?
- Have the views and preferences of the target population (patients, public, etc.) been sought?
- Have the target users of the guideline been clearly defined?

Domain 3: Rigour of Development: Using the Best Evidence to Inform Recommendations

- Is it clear how the evidence used to inform the document was searched for and selected? Was there a robust strategy of where to look for evidence and criteria for what to include/exclude?
- Are the strengths/limitations of the evidence used made clear, including acknowledging how the evidence sits within the recognised hierarchy of evidence? Is the evidence used current and relevant to the objectives/scope of the document?
- Are the recommendations of the document explicitly linked to the evidence? Have they been externally reviewed by experts prior to its publication?

- Were the health benefits, side-effects and risks considered in formulating the recommendations?
- Is it clear how the document will be updated to incorporate new evidence? Is there a process for reviewing the document?

Domain 4: Clarity of Presentation

- Is it clear what the purpose or intent of the recommendation(s) are?
- Are the key recommendations presented in a way that is easy to identify/ user friendly, e.g. summarised/in a box/table or flowchart? Are specific recommendations grouped together so that they are easy to find?
- Are the different options for management of the condition or health issue clearly presented (e.g. different client groups/different healthcare professionals)?
- Is it clear which population groups the recommendations apply to or any that they specifically *do not* apply to?

Domain 5: Applicability

- Are any client groups/care situations/clinical scenarios obviously missing from the recommendations?
- Is it clear what limitations/barriers/facilitators to applying the recommendations there might be, for example the need for training/ specialised equipment?
- Have any cost implications have been considered?
- Is there advice on how the recommendations can be applied in practice, e.g. summary documents/checklists/flowcharts?
- If applicable, have the outcome of pilot tests and lessons learned been presented in the document?
- Have monitoring/auditing criteria been presented, with advice as to the frequency of measurement and monitoring?

Domain 6: Competing/Conflicting Interests. Editorial Independence

- Have competing interests of guideline development group members been recorded and addressed?
- Is it clear how the development of the document was funded/who commissioned it? Is it clear that the recommendations were not influenced by any funding body?

Suggested reading at the end of this chapter provides more detail on the use of clinical guidelines in practice.

Reviewing the Literature to Find Evidence for Practice

Key sources of evidence for practice include research studies, the opinions of those considered experts in a field of practice and the lived experiences of patients and service users. This evidence is usually found in the published works of others, known as secondary sources.

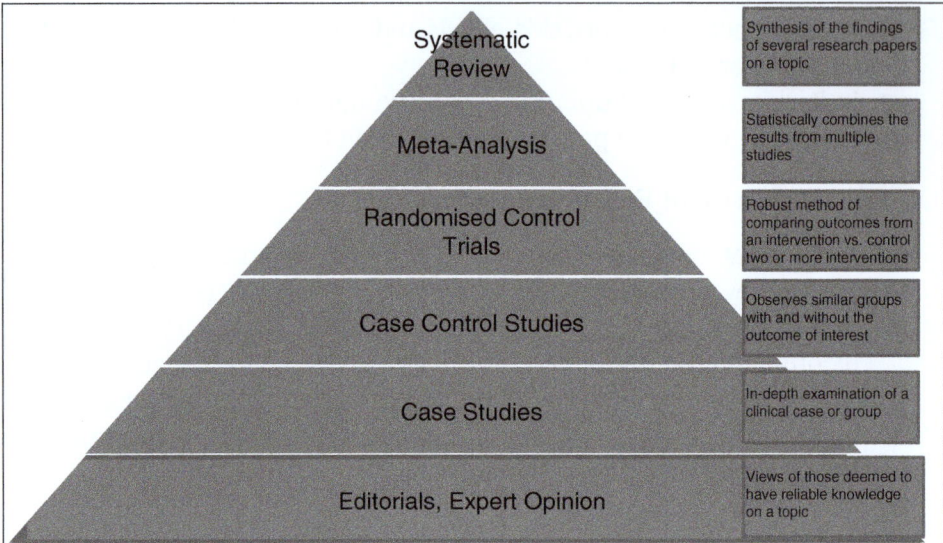

Figure 8.1: Hierarchy of evidence.

What Published Evidence Should I Look At?

Finding good-quality evidence to answer clinical questions can be daunting and it is tempting to think that anything that has been published must be true. However, some types of evidence are considered more trustworthy than others and there is an accepted hierarchy of published evidence. Picking and choosing to consider only some of the available evidence can lead to misrepresentation of knowledge and the best healthcare decisions are based on the synthesis of all the good-quality evidence available. This is why current, well-designed systematic reviews and meta-analyses that rigorously re-examine and reanalyse original study data are at the top of the hierarchy (Figure 8.1). Expert opinion and anecdotal experience are at the bottom of the hierarchy as they lack corroboration and transparency. This evidence is often specific to a particular local area and so may not be transferrable to your area of practice.

Reflective Activity

- In relation to the student question 'Why are parents and carers not bringing their children to our clinic for the MMR vaccination?', explore the original evidence published in *The Lancet* (Wakefield et al. 1988) that reported a link between the MMR vaccination and autism.
- Why do you think that this evidence was originally considered credible? What impact is this publication still having on the uptake of the MMR vaccination today?

Reading sources that may help you with this activity are included in the suggested reading section at the chapter end.

Finding Evidence Collated by Others

You may not feel competent to find good-quality evidence to review and searching for evidence takes time. There are a range of resources that provide access to collated published evidence for you. The NHS provides an evidence-based healthcare resource guide at: `https://libguides.sgul.ac.uk/ld.php?content_id=32001469`

Sources of Collated Evidence for Clinical Practice

- **NICE Evidence:** a good place to begin looking for evidence. This database aims to give easy access to a range of UK evidence-based resources online.
- **NICE Clinical Knowledge Summaries (CKS):** provide clinical presentations and patient scenarios to illustrate the current evidence base and practical guidance in respect of over 350 clinical topics.
- **Evidence-based Nursing:** searches a wide range of international healthcare journals of relevance to best nursing practice, focusing on the papers' key findings and implications for nursing.
- **Cochrane Library:** identifies systematic reviews and other high-quality reviews. It provides synthesis of the results and conclusions of primary studies in a particular field that meet robust standards of scientific method.
- **UpToDate and Dynamed:** these evidence-based clinical resources aim to provide clinical decision support to help answer clinical questions.

Searching the Published Literature

If you want to answer a specific question, rather than looking for evidence around a particular theme (such as a particular illness or treatment), you may need to undertake a focused look at the published literature using key words to narrow down your search. You will probably have some experience of this as part of your Foundation degree and will already appreciate that it is a systematic process requiring you to be clear about your question (to identify your key search words) and then look critically at the literature identified.

Nursing research and expert opinion tend to be published in academic journals. Looking at the hierarchy of evidence, you can see the sort of evidence you should be considering. It needs to be credible, reliable, relevant and up to date. The best evidence is likely to be published in journals that have a clear scope and robust processes for selecting the content and reviewing the quality of the material before publication.

It may be tempting to use Google Scholar for speed to search for articles, but this search engine has no clear strategy for selecting its 'scholarly' material which varies in quality and leaves you to decide which search results are suitable. Academic databases gather the contents of academic journals, allowing you to find published articles about a specific theme. They are particularly good if you want to combine two or more key words together. For example, the student asking a question about repositioning in order to reduce the risk of pressure ulcer in patients being cared for on a frail elderly ward might search for 'frail' AND 'elderly' AND 'pressure ulcers' AND 'repositioning' to find articles that address all concepts together. It can be helpful to search under alternative terms for key words, for example 'decubitus ulcer' as an alternative to 'pressure ulcer'.

Your university or Trust library will be a useful resource. Databases such as the British Nursing Index (BNI) are good places to start. The BNI has access to over 300 nursing and midwifery journals, containing details of English language publications from 1985, and it is updated monthly. Other databases include CINAHL (for nursing and allied health professionals) and MEDLINE (for more medical publications). These databases allow you to narrow your searches, for example by date and selecting peer-reviewed and full-text articles. Your clinical library can advise you further and may even help you undertake searches. Regularly scanning the content of key journals in your subject area will help you keep up to date with new evidence for practice.

The access management system Open Athens allows the use of one username and password to access a wide range of online resources, including full-text online journals, online books and the main healthcare databases in which you can search for information on your topic. You can also use your account to access important summaries of evidence and some e-learning.

Evaluating the Evidence That You Find

There is little point spending time and effort working with evidence that lacks credibility, as others may not engage with you and your work is unlikely to result in improved care. You need to be able to critically appraise evidence to be confident that current care or planned changes in practice have a sound rationale. Finding the best evidence to inform practice can be challenging, particularly with the ever-growing amount of material available.

The hierarchy of evidence provides a starting point for assessing evidence quality. The Critical Appraisal Skills Programme (CASP) checklists are freely available online and can help you perform critical appraisals for several different research methods. The checklists encourage you to consider the following questions.

- Is the study methodology sound?
- Are the results of the study valid?
- What are the results?
- Will the results help locally?

There is also an online guide on how to use the checklists at: https://casp-uk. net/casp-tools-checklists

Finding New Evidence for Practice

The main types of evidence used to answer clinical questions and develop the knowledge base for practice will now be considered in some detail. As you read about each type of evidence, think about how each one could be applied to question(s) that you have about clinical practice.

Evidence from Systematic Enquiry through Research

Research involves adding to what is already known by generating new knowledge, known as primary data, in an organised way; this is often called the research process. The NMC has highlighted the importance of ensuring that decisions about care and treatment consider what research has been shown to be most effective (NMC 2018a) (Standard 1.7). Nurses and NAs make up the largest staff group within the healthcare workforce and they have a key part to play in influencing what research questions are asked and how knowledge is shared and implemented into practice. As an NA, you may have the opportunity to be involved in carrying out research yourself, through increasing opportunities to work within clinical research nursing teams; you will also need to use evidence from the findings of others to inform your practice.

> **Reflective Activity**
>
> ■ Return to your earlier question relating to your area of practice.
> ■ Discuss the question with your colleagues. Have they thought about this question in their area of practice?
> ■ Is your question worded in a way that helps you focus on a search of the literature to help you find some answers? If not, think how you might reword it. What are your key words?

We will now look at different research methods.

Research Methods

The method used to carry out research depends on the question being asked and the type of information considered most appropriate to answer it. It also depends on the theoretical perspective taken by the researcher and the skills, resources, time and support they have. A broad question will need to be narrowed down to determine the research method and the type of data collected. A focused question considers the population group (e.g. type of patient, such as frail elderly); the area of interest or the problem (e.g. pressure ulcer development); any intervention (e.g. frequency of repositioning the patient); and any comparisons or outcomes (e.g. incidence and grading of pressure ulcer development).

Research methods are often divided into 'quantitative' and 'qualitative' depending on the kind of evidence (data) they generate.

Quantitative Methods

These methods tend to be used for questions that focus on causation, outcome and prognosis, often the What? and When? questions. This evidence is based on numbers, is measurable and tells us how many, how much or how often. Clinical research trials that test medical, surgical or behavioural interventions are the primary way that researchers determine if new forms of treatment or prevention are safe and effective. These studies usually collect numerical data that can be analysed statistically to show that outcomes are not just the result of chance.

Not all quantitative research is carried out in large clinical trials and it may be that your particular questions about practice could be best answered using a quantitative approach. Below are some examples from the questions that were asked by students, highlighting how they might be explored quantitatively. You can probably think of other ways of approaching each question.

Theme of Questions

- Effectiveness of hand hygiene measures in mental health inpatient settings compared to acute medical wards.
- Frequency of repositioning patients at risk of developing pressure ulcers on frail elderly wards.
- Choice of wound dressing in a surgical ward and in community settings.
- Uptake of the MMR vaccine.

Focused Questions

- Is there a difference in the number of hospital-acquired infections in mental health ward patients compared to those on medical wards?
- Does the length of time between repositioning patients on a frail elderly ward impact on the incidence of pressure ulcer development?
- Does the wound dressing used in my surgical ward promote wound healing more effectively than the wound dressing used in the community?
- Are there demographic differences between attenders and non-attenders for the MMR vaccine at our clinic?

Examples of Data That Could Be Collected

- Retrospective collection of the numbers of hospital-acquired infections in mental health and medical inpatient settings. These data could provide evidence of difference in hospital-acquired infections in two clinical settings.
- Correlate data from repositioning charts kept at the bedside with the incidence of pressure ulcer development. These data could provide evidence of a link between repositioning frequency and pressure ulcer development.
- Compare wound healing rates with similar patients in the community and on the surgical ward. These data could provide evidence that supports one type of dressing being more effective than another at promoting wound healing.
- Record demographic details of parent/carer and compare attenders to non-attenders for significant differences. These data could provide evidence for the significance of factors such as age, sex, education, employment and number of children.

Qualitative Methods

Questions that focus on exploring experiences and understanding Why? and How? are best answered with descriptive evidence based on interpretation. This type of research often finds evidence from practitioners and service users. The student questions could also be addressed using a qualitative approach and examples are highlighted below. You can probably think of other focused questions that you could ask.

Theme of Question

- Effectiveness of hand hygiene measures in mental health inpatient settings compared to acute medical wards.
- Frequency of repositioning patients at risk of developing pressure ulcers on frail elderly wards.
- Choice of wound dressing a surgical ward and in community settings.
- Uptake of the MMR vaccine.

Focused Questions

- What do nursing staff in mental health in patient settings consider to be the challenges in implementing our hand hygiene policy in practice?
- How do nurses working on our frail elderly ward determine the frequency of repositioning their patients?
- What do surgical ward nursing staff and those in community care settings think about the wound dressings they have available to use?
- Are there demographic differences between attenders and non-attenders for the MMR vaccine at our clinic?

Examples of Data That Could Be Collected

- Interviews with a sample of mental health inpatient unit nursing staff to ask about perceived challenges in cleaning their hands in accordance with policy. Evidence from key themes could include data around lack of awareness of the recommendations, challenging the recommendations, access to equipment, workload.
- Tape-recorded focus group discussion with nurses working on a frail elderly ward to explore the decisions that determine how frequently patients are turned. Evidence from key themes could include data around awareness of guidelines, risk assessment, environmental factors and patient choice.
- Interview surgical ward nursing staff and community nurses about their experiences with wound dressings. Evidence from key themes could include data around ease of applying the dressing, frequency of dressing change, cost, patient preference, perceived effectiveness for wound healing.
- Telephone survey with those who choose not to bring their child for vaccination to identify key themes. Evidence from key themes could include data around understanding of the vaccination, previous experience with vaccinations, family attitude and access to the surgery.

Sometimes questions are best answered through the evidence from a mixture of both quantitative and qualitative data. This is known as a mixed methods approach and can bring a broader perspective to the evidence.

It is beyond the scope of this chapter to go through all the different methods used in research and indeed, researchers tend to be experts only in research methods they have used themselves. There are many good resources available should you want to know more about the method of a particular research study that you come across (see the suggested reading at the chapter end).

Most NHS Trusts and other healthcare providers have research strategies highlighting areas of specialism in research and future research priorities.

Reflective Activity

- Have a look for your local research strategy. Is there any research being carried out in your clinical area? Are there any nursing research priorities?
- Find out if you are able to spend time in your local research office, with clinical research nurses or those undertaking research while in clinical practice roles.

Limitations of Systematic Research as a Source of Evidence to Inform Practice

While the structured and rigorous approach behind research might make it seem the most credible and robust source of evidence, a question that focuses on a small section of the patient or service user population (selected for age, sex, health status, etc.) may produce evidence that is not applicable to the wider population. Research topics are influenced by political agendas and financial priorities and not all aspects of care receive the same attention. Complex research methods and statistical analysis can make evidence inaccessible and difficult to understand and this can limit its application to practice.

Evidence from Clinical Expertise

Clinical expertise develops over time because of meaningful experience in a particular field of practice. It is framed by experience, knowledge and skills that are underpinned by theoretical knowledge. It has been recognised that nurses develop expertise in stages as they transition from being a novice (Benner 1984). You may feel that you are developing expertise as you spend more time in a particular clinical area.

Those considered experts may not be able to tell you how they came to be identified as such, although clinical expertise is often assumed because of an individual's job role – nurse specialists, for example. The role of expert is often endorsed through the behaviours of others who defer to particular individuals whenever decisions need to be made. Colleagues and service users may ask you questions because they think you know the answers and an important part of developing expertise is acknowledging the things that you do not know.

If you have a question about practice, you may seek the advice of those who you consider experts. Individuals you work with, peers working in similar clinical areas, those posting on online forums or presenting at conferences, as well as published authors, are all potential experts. As with all sources of evidence, it is important to be confident in the credibility and relevance of their information before using it as evidence to inform your own practice.

Evidence from Patient or Service User Experience, Preference and Values

The Standards of Proficiency for the NA role (NMC 2018a) state that 'the personal situation, characteristics, preferences and wishes of people, their families and carers need to be considered when providing care'. Your day-to-day practice will involve making decisions about care that considers the specific needs of individuals. These decisions will be based on the holistic assessment and care planning that help form the evidence for person-centred care (see Chapter 4 for more detail around person-centred care).

Patients and service users are often experts in their health and illness and will know what is normal for them and what is not. They are likely to get information from a range of sources and while they may not have a full understanding of their medical condition or the range of care options available, they will have a view about care that is effective and what makes a good-quality patient experience. As well as considering this within day-to-day care delivery, this personal knowledge can be captured as rich qualitative data in research studies that explore lived experiences.

The involvement of patients, carers, members of the public and communities is now an expected part of health research. Many healthcare settings actively recruit into clinical trials and as someone who works clinically, you may well be involved in discussions that support clinical research nurses in recruiting participants. Clinical research nurses are involved in receiving informed consent from prospective participants to take part in research. This is particularly relevant as the research often involves randomisation into particular treatment groups and/or a change in routine care or treatment. They also collect data from clinical records and conduct follow-up appointments. The have an important role in ensuring that patients are treated both ethically and safely throughout the research process, following the four principles of healthcare ethics.

The four principles of medical ethics were originally defined by Beauchamp and Childress in 1979.

- Respect for the patient's right to self-determination: to decide whether to take part in research.
- Beneficence: the duty to 'do good'.
- Non-maleficence: the duty to 'not do bad'.
- Justice: to treat all people equally and equitably.

Translating Evidence into Practice

If you have asked a question about practice and found what you consider to be the best evidence to answer it, the next stage is to implement this evidence into care delivery in order to improve the quality of care provided. This might involve adapting the information and advice that you currently give to service users. It requires presenting evidence in a way that is meaningful and user friendly for those who need to use it.

Reflective Activity

Think about how you would use credible evidence about the MMR vaccination to support your answers to the following questions that you might be asked by parents or carers.

- I have heard that there is a link between the MMR jab and autism – is this true?
- I would like my child to wait until they are older to have the MMR jab. I think they would cope with it better. What do you think?
- Why should my child have the MMR jab if other children around here are not having it?

The suggested reading at the chapter end may help with your answers.

New evidence may suggest that current practice needs to be updated or modified. It may be necessary to introduce completely new ways of working. This will mean that practices that have been established for some time will need to be stopped and this can lead to resistance to change. Practices such as egg white and oxygen for pressure ulcer care and gauze wicks soaked in a solution of lime to promote wound healing were once considered best practice. The evidence-based practices you champion today will be replaced as care evolves and new evidence is found.

To change practice successfully requires the right culture, the right leadership, capability in interpreting and implementing evidence and engaging staff and patients in evidence-based policy and practice (NHS England and NHS Improvement 2020). The difficulty in relating evidence to clinical practice is sometimes called the 'theory–practice gap'

Reflective Activity

- Look for an example of where credible evidence is being used to support something that you do in your clinical practice. What factors do you think have influenced the use of this evidence in your area of practice?

The suggested reading at the chapter end provides more information on the translation of evidence into nursing practice. Students used this as guided reading and produced the following SWOT analysis of key themes.

The evidence

Strengths	Weaknesses
Good quality, relevant, current	Lack of evidence on the topic
Consistent findings	Not easy to access, poor quality, not applicable
Clearly presented and accessible	Confusing and unclear findings

Organisational factors

Opportunities	Threats
A culture where evidence-based practice is championed and supported	The topic is not seen as a priority (local and political agendas)
Practical ways to encourage awareness about the evidence such as journal clubs, shared decision making, conference attendance	Ineffective leadership, lack of support, reluctance to change the status quo
Opportunities for taking part in all aspects of evidence-based practice – working with research nurses, policy development, service evaluation and audit	Not valuing evidence-based practice and/or thinking it is other people's responsibility
	Lack of resources – time, finances
Opportunities for developing skills and confidence – continuing education, library support, research outreach	Not having the knowledge or skills to find and then interpret/ appraise the evidence
Opportunities for sharing ideas and support with dissemination of evidence (e.g. publication)	Not having the skills, authority or permission to make changes

The development of knowledge and understanding from evidence is an evolutionary process and takes time. Taking the example of the NA, initial questions about the role were addressed through personal opinion and individual experiences. It has taken time for the role to be explored using systematic research. However, the findings from such studies are now being published and there is an emerging knowledge base for the NA role that has the potential to influence its development in practice. The suggested reading at the chapter end includes some of these publications.

Clinical Decision Making

There is not much point knowing what the best evidence tells us we ought to be doing if this evidence is not being used consistently in practice. The NA is expected to make evidence-based decisions and solve problems (NMC 2018a). Within the realities of day-to-day working, the opportunities and challenges you face in being confident that your practice is evidence based are complex. Clinical decisions involve a complex interplay between sources of evidence and specific service user and environmental circumstances. Making sound clinical decisions will involve developing the knowledge, skills and confidence to champion care that is known to be safe and effective. While you will be working under the supervision of a registered nurse, as an accountable practitioner, you will be required to justify the care that you give. You will need to be able to challenge preconceptions and poor practice and defend care that is evidence based.

Reflective Activity

Students have said that they find it difficult to challenge practice they encounter that is not based on best practice or sound evidence. For example, some have said that they feel unsure what to do if they see colleagues not cleaning their hands between caring for patients. Think about what you would do in this situation.

Monitoring Evidence in Practice

Service Evaluation

It takes time for the evidence generated from systematic research methods to be translated into local practice. When organisations need prompt answers, service evaluation is used to capture 'real-time' data to measure or define current practice quickly. It is an approach used to understand the value of a service and highlight the extent to which it is meeting its aims.

Those in nursing roles are increasingly involved in service evaluation as their clinical position makes them well placed to evaluate practice and be involved in acting on the evidence in order to develop practice. Service evaluation often seeks feedback on the experiences of service users. It differs from pure scientific research in its practical nature, generating findings that can be used as evidence to develop tangible changes in practice to improve the quality of care delivery and inform local decision making. For example, you could ask service users to complete a questionnaire on their perceptions of the hand hygiene practices of those caring for them. The results could be used to inform training for healthcare practitioners in your organisation. A GP practice might undertake a survey to evaluate what parents and carers thought about the information they were given about the MMR vaccination. The findings could be used to improve the information provided.

Clinical Audit

Clinical audit is a quality improvement tool that is used to monitor, assess and improve the quality of care in a clinical environment. It is a cyclical process that involves measuring an outcome or process and comparing this to current evidence or best practice. It is often policy or guideline recommendations that are audited. Audit data need to be acted on to inform changes designed to improve care quality.

Reflective Activity

Thinking about the student question on hand hygiene ...

■ Is there a hand hygiene policy/guideline in your clinical area? If so, have a go at reviewing it against the domains of the Agree Reporting Checklist (Brouwers et al. 2016). What do you conclude about your policy/guideline as a source of evidence-based recommendations for your practice? The suggested reading at the chapter end may help you with this.

- In your clinical area, do you monitor to see if hand hygiene recommendations are carried out in practice? Is there an audit? If so, consider the following.
  - Where is the audit carried out?
  - Who carries out the audit?
  - When does the audit take place and how often?
  - What is audited? What data are collected?
  - How is the information collated, presented and disseminated?
  - Are you involved in the audit process? If not, why not?
  - Is there a clear link between the audit and the policy/guideline recommendations?
  - What if anything is the impact of the audit? Does it lead to a change in practice/improved quality of care?
  - What would you change/do differently to make the audit more effective?

You may want to undertake similar critical reviews of other audits undertaken in your area of practice. Think about what you would do with your findings.

The suggested reading at the chapter end provides more detail on clinical audit.

Chapter Summary

This chapter has explored the significance of evidence-based practice from the perspective of the NA. It has highlighted ways in which you may be involved in finding and reviewing evidence which can be used to inform clinical practice. You have been encouraged to think about the application of key components of evidence-based practice to your particular role and clinical situation. The challenge is to continue to be curious through the use of evidence that promotes quality, avoids harm and makes considered use of resources. Using your knowledge and experience to make evidence-based decisions and solve problems will help you realise your potential to positively influence the experience of patients and service users.

References

Avery, M., Westwood, G., and Richardson, A. (2021). Enablers and barrier to progressing a clinical academic career in nursing, midwifery and allied health professions: a cross-sectional survey. *Journal of Clinical Nursing* 31 (3–4): 406–416.

Beauchamp, T.L. and Childress, J.F. (1979). *Principles of Biomedical Ethics*. Oxford: Oxford University Press.

Benner, P. (1984). *From Novice to Expert, Excellence and Power in Clinical Nursing Practice*. Menlo Park: Addison-Wesley.

Brouwers, C., Kerkvliet, K., Spithoff, K., and AGREE Next Steps Consortium (2016). The AGREE Reporting Checklist: a tool to improve reporting of clinical practice guidelines. *BMJ* 352: 1152.

Cassidy, C.E., Harrison, M.B., Godfrey, C. et al. (2021). Use and effects of implementation strategies for practice guidelines in nursing: a systematic review. *Implementation Science* 16 (1): 1–29.

Department of Health and Social Care, Executive Office (Northern Ireland), Scottish Government and Welsh Government (2021). The Future of Clinical Research Delivery 2022–2025. www.gov.uk/government/publications/the-future-of-uk-clinical-research-delivery

European Society of Cardiology (ESC) (2023). 2023 ESC guidelines for the management of acute coronary syndromes. www.escardio.org/Guidelines/Clinical-Practice-Guidelines/Acute-Coronary-Syndromes-ACS-Guidelines

Guyatt, G.H. (1991). Evidence-based medicine. *ACP Journal Club* 114 (2): A–16.

Haywood, J. (1975). *Information: A Prescription against Pain*. London: Royal College of Nursing.

Health Education England (2015). *Raising the Bar: Shape of Caring: A Review of the Future Education and Training of Registered Nurses and Care Assistants*. London: Health Education England.

HMSO (1972). Report of the Committee on Nursing. Chairman Professor Ada Briggs. London: HMSO.

Intercollegiate Stroke Working Party (2023). National Clinical Guideline for stroke for the UK and Ireland. www.strokeguideline.org

Kitson, A., Harvey, G., Gifford, W. et al. (2021). How nursing leaders promote evidence-based practice implementation at point-of-care: a four-country exploratory study. *Journal of Advanced Nursing* 77 (5): 2447–2457.

Medical Research Council (1944). Clinical trial of patulin in the common cold. *Lancet* 2: 373–375.

Muir Gray, J.A. (1997). *Evidence-Based Health Care: How to Make Health Policy and Management Decisions*. London: Churchill Livingstone.

National Institute for Health and Care Excellence (NICE) (2014) Developing NICE guidelines: the manual. www.nice.org.uk/process/pmg20

NHS England (2019). The NHS Long Term Plan. www.longtermplan.nhs.uk/publication/nhs-long-term-plan

NHS England and NHS Improvement (2020). Leading the acceleration of evidence into practice: a guide for executive nurses. www.england.nhs.uk/wp-content/uploads/2020/03/leading-the-acceleration-of-evidence-into-practice-guide.pdf

Nursing and Midwifery Council (NMC) (2018a). Standards of proficiency for registered nursing associates. www.nmc.org.uk/standards/standards-for-nursing-associates/standards-of-proficiency-for-nursing-associates/

Nursing and Midwifery Council (NMC) (2018b). The code. www.nmc.org.uk/standards/code/

Royal College of Nursing (RCN) (2023). *New Definition of Nursing: Background research and rationale*. London: RCN.

Royal College of Nursing (RCN) (2024). *The Royal College of Nursing Research Strategy: 2024–2027 Promoting Leadership, Voice and Visibility of Nurses in Research*. London: RCN.

Royal College of Nursing (RCN) (1996). *Clinical Effectiveness*. London: RCN.

Sackett, D.L., Rosenberg, W.M., Gray, J.A. et al. (1996). Evidence based medicine: what it is and what it isn't. *BMJ* 312 (7023): 71.

Stockwell, F. (1972). *The Unpopular Patient*. London: Royal College of Nursing.

Wakefield, A.J., Murch, S.H., Anthony, A. et al. (1988). Ileal-lymphoid-nodular hyperplasia, non-specific colitis, and pervasive developmental disorder in children. *Lancet* 351: 637–641.

World Health Organization (WHO) (2022). Global competency framework. www.who.int/news/item/19-07-2022-global-competency-framework

Further Reading

Evidence-based practice

Kumah, E.A., McSherry, R., Bettany-Saltikov, J. and Van Schaik, P. (2022). Evidence-informed practice: simplifying and applying the concept for nursing students and academics. *British Journal of Nursing*, 31(6), 322–330.

Owens, M. Adams, J. Rogers, P. Smith, H. and Welsh, V. (2024). *Understanding Evidence-Based Practice for Nursing Associates*. London: Learning Matters.

Research methods

Harvey, M. and Land, L. (2021). *Research Methods for Nurses and Midwives: Theory and Practice*. London: Sage.

Health Research Authority (2022). Is my study research? Defining research. www.hra-decisiontools.org.uk/research/

Polit, D. and Beck, C. (2020). *Essentials of Nursing Research: Appraising Evidence for Nursing Practice*. Philadelphia: Lippincott Williams and Wilkins.

Use of clinical guidelines in practice

National Institute for Health and Care Excellence (NICE) (2018). *Principles of Putting Evidence Based guidance into Practice*. London: National Institute for Health and Care Excellence.

Redley, B., Douglas, T., Hoon, L., White, K. and Hutchinson, A. (2022). Nursing guidelines for comprehensive harm prevention strategies for adult patients in acute hospitals: an integrative review and synthesis. *International Journal of Nursing Studies*, 127, 104178.

Spoon, D., Rietbergen, T., Huis, A. et al. (2020). Implementation strategies used to implement nursing guidelines in daily practice: a systematic review. *International Journal of Nursing Studies*, 111, 103748.

Patients as sources of evidence for practice

Ellis, P. (2023). Working with others to achieve evidence based care. In: Ellis, P. (ed.) *Evidence Based Practice in Nursing*. London: Sage, pp. 106–116.

Greenhalgh, T., Hinton, L., Finlay, T., Macfarlane, A., Fahy, N., Clyde, B. and Chant, A. (2019). Frameworks for supporting patient and public involvement in research: systematic review and co-design pilot. *Health Expectations*, 22(4), 785–801.

Jones, M. and Pietilä, I. (2020). Personal perspectives on patient and public involvement – stories about becoming and being an expert by experience. *Sociology of Health & Illness*, 42(4), 809–824.

Factors influencing the translation of evidence into nursing practice

Hare, N. and Whitehouse, C. (2022). Engaging with research: practical advice for nurses at every level. *Nursing Standard* 37 3, 30–34.

Kerr, H. and Rainey, D. (2021). Addressing the current challenges of adopting evidence-based practice in nursing. *British Journal of Nursing*, 30(16), 970–974.

Clinical decision making

Cleary-Holdforth, J. and Leufer T. (2023). Using evidence for decision making. In: K. Holland and D. Roberts (eds) *Understanding Decision Making in Nursing Practice*. London: Sage, pp. 41–71.

Standing, M. (2023). Clinical decision making in evidence based nursing. In: Ellis P (ed.) *Evidence-Based Practice in Nursing*. London: Sage, pp. 124–151.

Clinical audit

Johnston, G., Crombie, I.K., Alder, E.M., Davies, H.T.O. and Millard, A. (2000). Reviewing audit: barriers and facilitating factors for effective clinical audit. *BMJ Quality and Safety*, 9(1), 23–36.

Peate, I. (2021). Clinical audit. In: Peate I (ed.) *The Nursing Associate at a Glance*. Chichester: Wiley Blackwell, pp. 120–121.

Service evaluation

Forde-Johnston, C. (2023). Service evaluation in healthcare explained using practice examples. www.youtube.com/watch?v=lySLgdKWlo0

Hand hygiene

Dickens, G.L., Goko, C. and Ryan, E. (2020). Nurses' attitudes and perceptions towards hand hygiene in mental health and medical inpatient settings: comparative, cross-sectional study. *Issues in Mental Health Nursing*, 41(11), 1011–1018.

Gould, D., Purssell, E., Jeanes, A., Drey, N., Chudleigh, J. and McKnight, J. (2022). The problem with 'my five moments for hand hygiene'. *BMJ Quality and Safety*, 31(4), 322–326.

Hillier, M. (2020). Using effective hand hygiene practice to prevent and control infection. *Nursing Standard* 35, 45–50.

Wound dressings and wound care

Gillespie, B.M., Walker, R.M., McInnes, E. et al. (2020). Preoperative and postoperative recommendations to surgical wound care interventions: a systematic meta-review of Cochrane reviews. *International Journal of Nursing Studies*, 102, 103486.

Lumbers, M. (2020). New tools in wound care to support evidence-based best practice. *British Journal of Community Nursing*, 25(3), S26–S29.

Powell K, Pujji OJS and Jeffery S. (2021). Wound healing: what is the NICE guidance from the UK? *Journal of Wound Care*. 30(3): 172–182.

Prevention of pressure ulcers

Alshahrani, B., Sim, J. and Middleton, R. (2021). Nursing interventions for pressure injury prevention among critically ill patients: a systematic review. *Journal of Clinical Nursing*, 30(15–16), 2151–2168.

Avsar, P., Moore, Z., Patton, D., O'Connor, T., Budri, A.M. and Nugent, L. (2020). Repositioning for preventing pressure ulcers: a systematic review and meta-analysis. *Journal of Wound Care*, 29(9), 496–508.

MMR vaccine uptake

Hill, M.C., Salmon, D., Chudleigh, J. and Aitken, L.M. (2021). Practice nurses' perceptions of their immunization role and strategies used to promote measles, mumps, and rubella vaccine uptake in 2014–2018: a qualitative study. *Journal of Advanced Nursing*, 77(2), 948–956.

Oxford Vaccine Group (2024). MMR vaccination (measles, mumps and rubella vaccine). https://vaccineknowledge.ox.ac.uk/mmr-vaccine

Torracinta L, Tanner R and Vanderslott S. (2021). MMR vaccine attitude and uptake research in the United Kingdom: a critical review. *Vaccines* 9(4): 402.

The nursing associate role

Lucas, G., Brook, J., Thomas, T., Daniel, D., Ahmet, L. and Salmon, D. (2021). Healthcare professionals' views of a new second-level nursing associate role: a qualitative study exploring early implementation in an acute setting. *Journal of Clinical Nursing*, 30(9–10), 1312–1324.

Robertson, S., King, R., Taylor, B. et al. (2024). Development of the nursing associate role in community and primary care settings across England. *Nursing Open*, 11(3), e2131.

Thurgate, C. and Griggs, C. (2023). Nursing associates 6 years on: a review of the literature. *Journal of Clinical Nursing*, 32(17–18), 6028–6036.

9 Supporting Learners: The Role of the Nursing Associate

Annabel Coulson

University Hospitals of Leicester NHS Trust, Leicester, UK

Introduction

As you draw towards the end of your pre-registration programme, you will need to consider what it will mean to transition and become a registrant; how will this change your level of responsibility both in terms of your accountability to care for your patients and your responsibility to support others to learn and develop their skills. This chapter will explore this changing role in relation to the support and supervision of learners; you will need to reflect critically on your experience as a learner to prepare yourself for your future role. This chapter will contain useful resources for both the student nursing associate (NA) and new registrant.

As a student NA, you may have previously worked within a healthcare setting before commencing the programme; this chapter will draw on these previous experiences while being equally relevant if you are new to care within this role. As a healthcare assistant (HCA) or healthcare support worker (HCSW), you may have worked alongside a range of different learners but had little involvement in their formal education and preparation for their role. You should not, however, underestimate the amount of support you gave to learners, almost without realising, as you shared your experience and understanding with them. In your new role as a NA, you will be responsible for supporting learners and making a judgement as to their ability to meet the expectations of the programme of study they are engaged in. You will be expected to support, teach and assess against the relevant standards and provide evidence for the decisions you make with regard to assessment, and you will be answerable for these decisions to the regulatory body, the Nursing and Midwifery Council (NMC 2018a).

The Nursing Associate: Stepping into Practice, First Edition. Edited by Annabel Coulson.
© 2025 John Wiley & Sons Ltd. Published 2025 by John Wiley & Sons Ltd.

In order to meet the requirements of this part of your role, you need to understand and be able to apply the relevant NMC Standards; in the case of supporting learners, this is the NMC Standards for student support and supervision (NMC 2018c). This chapter aims to develop your understanding and application of these standards and support you to relate this to your role.

Aims of This Chapter

By the end of this chapter, you will:

- have a greater understanding of the learning environment and the importance of developing an effective culture for learning
- understand the role of the NA in supporting others to learn through practice
- develop an understanding of the NMC Standards for student supervision and assessment and the role of the NA
- develop an understanding of the importance of effective feedback to improve standards.

Related NMC Standards

Platform 4

4.6 Demonstrate the ability to monitor and review the quality of care delivered, providing challenge and constructive feedback, when an aspect of care has been delegated to others.

4.7 Support, supervise and act as a role model to NA students, HCSWs and those new to care roles, review the quality of the care they provide, promoting reflection and providing constructive feedback.

4.8 Contribute to team reflection activities, to promote improvements in practice and services.

NMC Standards of Student Support and Supervision

What are NMC Standards and why are they important?

The NMC will soon become your regulatory body and it is important that you understand how it sets and maintains the Standards for all educational programmes; you can find more information about the work of the NMC here: www.nmc.org.uk/about-us/our-role

The NMC is responsible for ensuring that only nurses, midwives and NAs who have the right knowledge, skills and behaviours to provide safe, effective and compassionate care are able to register and practise using these titles; this is aimed at ensuring public protection. When supporting learners, you will have a vital role in ensuring that effective assessments safeguard against those who are not able to provide person-centred care gaining access to the register.

Reflective Activity

- Consider for a moment the impact of this in relation to your role and level of accountability. As you work through this chapter, you might want to reflect on students and learners you have come across in practice.
- Take some time to read the NMC Standards for student support and supervision available at: www.nmc.org.uk/standards-for-education-and-training/standards-for-student-supervision-and-assessment

Reflective Activity

- Identify the different roles of practice assessor, practice supervisor and academic assessor. What has been your experience of these roles and the support provided? Reflecting on your own experience will help you to consider how you are going to support learners in the future.

These standards replaced mentors with practice supervisors (PS) and practice assessors (PA) with the aim of reducing the subjectivity associated with the support of learners (Duffy and Gillies 2018).

In practice, learners must be supervised by a registered professional who:

- upholds public protection
- provides inclusive, tailored learning experiences
- gives feedback
- contributes to decisions on assessment and progression
- raises concerns where necessary.

There are two key roles identified in the NMC Standards: the assessor, both academic and practice, and the practice supervisor. It is important to understand the fundamental differences between them and how they support the more objective approach the NMC was aiming for when it replaced the mentor role.

Assessors make judgements using the evidence a learner presents to them. This evidence might come from observed practice, through reflective accounts which have been verified by a practice supervisor or through testimony of other members of the team, patients or service users. The learner is responsible for gathering this evidence to provide enough information for the practice assessor to formulate a judgement.

Practice assessors must have:

- NMC registration with appropriate equivalent experience for the student's programme. As a NA, you can be a practice assessor for a student NA when you have been sufficiently prepared for the role in line with your organisation's policies or guidelines. You will usually have sufficient knowledge and skills at the end of your programme to be a practice supervisor, which we will explore later. Additional training is often given to ensure practice assessors (PA) understand their accountability regarding assessment. Pre-registration student nurses must be assessed by a PA who is a registered nurse

- the ability to conduct assessments to confirm that the student has achieved the requisite proficiencies and outcomes; to be able to conduct an effective assessment, a PA must have a good understanding of the programme of study
- an understanding of student's learning and achievement in theory.

Practice assessors work in partnership with the academic assessor regarding student progression. This means that there should be regular engagement between both practice and academic assessors and tripartite discussions with the student, particularly when any concerns have been identified.

The *academic assessor* must have an appropriate teaching qualification. They need an in-depth understanding of the programme of study and should be able to discuss both practice and academic progression and support both the student and the assessor to link these and ensure application to practice of taught theory. The aim of this inclusive process is to increase the positive relationship between the university and practice and provide the PA with support.

Assessment decisions are informed by feedback from practice supervisors, amongst other evidence presented by the learner as identified earlier.

Practice supervisors must have registration with a professional regulatory body, for example the NMC or the Health and Care Professionals Council (HCPC). This could be a physiotherapist or occupational therapist and learners may work with several practice supervisors with whom they can gather evidence to present to the PA. It is usual to have a small number of named practice supervisors such as NAs or registered nurses with whom the learner works regularly, to offer some consistency.

Learners must also be aware of their responsibility towards their own learning and must engage in their supervision and assessment in practice and must be:

- prepared for and have a sound understanding of the proficiencies they need to achieve
- aware of their responsibilities for completion of practice documentation
- aware of the person they should speak to in the practice area if they have concerns
- actively encouraged to seek out practice supervisors to support their learning and encourage feedback to be recorded in their Practice Assessment Documentation (PADs)
- made aware of their nominated PA at the beginning of the placement.

Experiences of Student Nursing Associates: Lessons Learnt

As you approach registration and start to consider your role as a practice supervisor and practice assessor, you should reflect on the positive or negative aspects of the supervision you have received. There is an increasing evidence base relating to the experiences of learners (King et al. 2020; Dainty et al. 2021). In 2024 the title 'trainee' NA was replaced with 'student' to recognise the importance of supporting learners within the practice setting and establishing a learning culture. You might want to reflect on these and the following points which reflect the experiences students have shared with the author; as a student you may have experienced this yourself.

- Lack of understanding of the role and the impact this has had on the learning experience.
- Practice supervisors and assessors who do not seem to value the role; lack of perceived value in the role by senior staff.
- Lack of protected learning time.

The Learning Environment

The learning environment is defined as the area in which learning takes place within the practice setting. The NMC requires educational institutions to determine, monitor and ensure the quality of the learning environment in which learners should be supported to develop the required skills and knowledge for their programme (NMC 2018a). As a student or an NA, you may have been employed in your main 'learning environment' before commencing the programme; depending on how your programme of study was devised, it may have been an important aspect of your early days on the programme to re-establish yourself as a learner rather than a HCA or HCSW. When supervising learners in any setting, it is important that you understand their background and we will explore this in more detail later. The term 'placement' will be used to define any learning environment used as an experience; this may be a base area or a specific experience you have undertaken as part of your programme. We will discuss later the importance of getting to know your learner and the experiences that have influenced their development.

The NMC states that all learners 'should be given the opportunity to learn and provide care across a range of different learning environments that will enable them to meet their learning outcomes and experience the variety of care situations for a diverse population'. Student NAs must experience a range of placements, or learning opportunities, that enable the integration of theory to practice across the life course; this includes 'in the home', 'close to home' and 'in hospital' (NMC 2018a). Students will also have some experience in all nursing 'fields of practice' including adult, child, learning disabilities and mental health environments; this range of experiences sets the NA programme apart from pre-registration nursing when students will predominantly experience placements which align to the field of nursing being studied for.

The NA programme is generic and transferable across fields of practice. As a student NA, you should embrace these different experiences to gain skills that you can transfer to all settings and recognise that people with a physical health concern may also have underlying mental health problems. As a generic practitioner, you have been provided with the skills and knowledge to recognise and support all service users in any setting. Areas that can provide a learning environment include hospitals, community nursing teams, inpatient centres, prisons, outpatient departments, GP centres; anywhere in which care is managed or delivered can provide a valuable learning experience with the right support from practice assessors and practice supervisors. All placements must have an educational audit to ensure that learners are safe and able to access appropriate support.

Depending on how programmes are devised, learners may spend more time in one area, which may be called the 'base' or 'hub', and attend placements elsewhere for shorter periods; these may be termed 'alternative' or 'spoke' placements.

Reflecting on your experience, how were your placement experiences arranged? How did this impact on your learning experience in each area as you progressed through the programme?

Student NAs have evaluated their early experiences on the NA programme, and understanding how these experiences have affected as individuals may give you some insight into the effect of a poor understanding of learning needs, which can be considered as you develop in your own role (Vanson and Beckett 2018).

SLOT Analysis of a Learning Environment

Depending on the structure of your programme, consider one of your placements or your main area of work if you were based there as a learner and explore this environment in more detail; what are the strengths and limitations, what opportunities exist to improve things, and what are the threats that might prevent the learning experience from being a positive one? Fill in the table below to reflect your conclusions.

Strengths	Limitations
Opportunities	**Threats**

Understanding the learning environment in this way can help you to make the most of the opportunities available both for you as a learner and for the future learners that you will support; you will be able to address the limitations and threats proactively rather than reactively to create a positive experience. When considering the strengths, ensure that you consider the wider nursing team and multidisciplinary team and how they can support you to maximise the opportunities available.

Learning in Practice

Depending on how a programme is managed, either through an apprenticeship or through a traditional university-based Foundation degree, there may be distinct differences in how learning in practice is managed. It is important that as a learner, you are aware of and understand these differences and as a practice supervisor, you consider the type of learner you are supporting; bear this in mind when you 'get to know your learner' as detailed later in this chapter.

Most NA programmes are delivered through an apprenticeship which means that students will undertake a mixture of 'protected learning' or 'off the job' hours and 'on the job'. 'Off the job' hours include both theory time, in the classroom, and protected learning time in practice; you may hear this called supernumerary time. Protected learning time should be detailed in the curriculum and is managed differently according to the programme; alternative 'spoke' placements in most programmes will be protected and you may also have some protected learning in your base placement. This protected learning time means that as a trainee, you are not included in the workforce numbers, and you can undertake specific experiences to complement your overall aims. You might, for example, visit different areas to see the patient journey, you might spend time with specialist teams or with other members of the MDT. In alternative 'spoke' placements, you will be unfamiliar with the setting and will need more direct supervision with all aspects of care delivery. As a practice supervisor supporting someone in an alternative placement, you will need to understand their experience and we will revisit this later in the chapter.

During 'on the job' hours you, or your learner, would be expected to contribute to the normal management of the area and this may include roles you are familiar with as a HCA/HCSW; you will, however, need to look at opportunities to develop skills, such as medication administration, supporting MDT plans and working with the medical team to understand the care for your patients. You will start to think critically about the care you are delivering and apply your knowledge with a more questioning approach; you should feel safe to ask questions and you should encourage your learners to question care in a proactive way. We will explore the importance of a positive learning culture on the feeling of psychological safety particularly around questioning approaches to care.

If you look at the evaluations of early implementation of the role, you will note that many students felt that this protected learning time was often eroded as a result of pressures within the workplace (Vanson and Beckett 2018; King et al. 2020). You may have had this experience as a learner, and it is important that you reflect on what this has meant for you during your programme; moving forward, you are in an ideal position to advocate for your learner and ensure that they are getting the experiences they need.

You may also act as a practice supervisor to a student nurse, and it is important to understand how their experience may differ; university-based pre-registration programmes require student nurses to be supernumerary while in the practice setting. Supernumerary status was mandated with the advent of Project 2000 in 1992 and all subsequent revisions to the education of pre-registration nursing students have maintained this approach (NMC 2018a). Having a greater understanding of some of the differences in education for nurses and NAs will allow you to gain insight into some of the comments made in the above evaluations relating to the priority apparently given to student nurses. As a practice supervisor, you will be ideally situated to ensure that all learners gain the type of experience and access to opportunities they need to feel confident (Henderson and Eaton 2013).

Review your SLOT analysis and consider the different types of learners in your learning environment. How are the opportunities affected by different understanding of the needs of learners? Does the learning environment facilitate and promote learning?

We will now explore the impact of a learning culture on the learning environment.

Learning Cultures

A learning culture exists when experienced staff can share knowledge and demonstrate good practice, providing the learner with time to question, practise and reflect on skills. A learning culture requires leadership which positively encourages openness and fosters trust; all members of the team should feel safe to question and challenge practice in order to enhance care (Henderson et al. 2011). Learning cultures are discussed in relation to a range of circumstances, for example the lessons learnt as a result of the enquiry into care at Mid Staffordshire hospitals (Francis 2013) or more recently the Ockendon Report into maternity services (Department of Health and Social Care and Independent Maternity Review 2022). A learning culture exists when there is no blame for mistakes, they can be openly discussed and as a result learning can take place. If you relate this to your learning experience and the experience you will give to the learners you are supporting, there is a need to allow a learner to question practice and to make mistakes; effective supervision will ensure that patient safety is maintained. Levels of supervision may mean that you prevent a learner from continuing with an action which may impact on the safety of your patients or service users. Managing this situation effectively will ensure that the learner gains from this experience and does not lose confidence (Levett-Jones et al. 2009).

Reflective Activity

- Critically reflect on your learning environment; is there a positive culture for learning and do people feel psychologically safe to make mistakes and learn from them?
- What is your responsibility if there is not a positive learning culture?
- When you meet a learner for the first time, how can you show them that a positive learning culture exists?

These activities encourage you to think critically about the environments you have experienced and how you will develop the support you provide to others.

The NMC Code states that a learning culture is required to ensure that the safety of people is prioritised; this includes carers, students and educators (NMC 2018b). Ensure that you check the Code as you approach registration to consider all aspects of your role, including your role in supporting others.

A positive learning culture:	A poor learning culture lacks:
Encourages	Acknowledgement of individual skills
Challenges	Understanding of learning aims
Helps to develop creative solutions	Interest in supporting others

A poor learning culture can lead to feelings of insecurity, including feeling bullied, can result in difficulties recruiting and retaining staff and staff may feel reluctant to speak out when they have concerns about care.

It is important that you remember not only the positive role models but also those who did not demonstrate a positive example of support and encouragement as you will alter your practice as much in response to this as you will to emulate someone you admire. A learning culture is not reliant on the ability and support of one individual but rather on the environment and all those within it; this requires positive leadership and collaboration within the team.

Now, more than ever, it is important that we develop a positive culture for learning – there are more people leaving the NHS than ever before and we need to support new learners and encourage them to want to come and work in this area when they complete their relevant programme. If you consider the number of times someone has highlighted poor staffing as a reason for giving a poor learning experience, does this make sense? We need staff, therefore we need the learner and we should ensure that they have a good experience and learn the knowledge, skills and behaviours they need to become a future professional or healthcare worker.

We have looked at the learning environment and the learning culture, both of which affect how you are able to support an individual.

Supporting Learners

Think about what a learner will need to know about an area when they arrive.

- What might they want to know before they arrive? Is any preparatory reading sent out? Who is responsible in your area for the overall learner experience?
- How will you know that this is relevant to them?
- What conversation would you have with your learner on arrival?

Earlier, you looked at the learning environment and developed a better understanding of the learning culture particularly in your own area; there are factors which will both support and inhibit learning.

Factors which support learning	Factors which inhibit learning
Feeling welcomed	Learners having to compete for experiences
Friendly staff	Being delegated menial tasks that do not challenge
Supervisors who are familiar with the learners' programme, aims and outcomes	The placement being too busy to enable opportunities to practise
Supervision from registered staff	Staff not interested in supervising learners
Diverse learning experiences	Unfriendly staff
Peer support from other learners	Students who are not actively engaged in their learning

While the learning environment and learning culture play an important role in supporting learning, as a practice supervisor you also need to be aware of factors internal to the learner themselves that may impact on their ability to learn within a placement area.

- Lack of self-belief
- Poor motivation/self-esteem
- Stress/tiredness/anxiety/illness, etc.
- Previous educational experiences, conditioning passive pedagogical approach
- Learning difference, e.g. dyslexia

Learners also have external pressures which may affect their learning and ability to engage with practice. However, you are not able to resolve all these issues and should be aware of support available from the educational institute. As a practice supervisor, it is important that you work collaboratively to minimise the impact of internal and external concerns on the overall learning experience.

- Time pressures/workload
- Family commitments, etc.
- Personality clash between learner and assessor/supervisor

Importance of Your Learners' Experience

You all have a range of experiences. You may have been in healthcare for some time and built up a network of peers and support systems. You may have experienced a lack of support within your practice, you may have experienced challenge or you may have been inspired by role models who gave you confidence in your own practice and supported your learning.

Whatever experience you have, professional and personal, this will impact on how you support others. You need to ensure that you are aware of this and reflect on how this experience may impact on you and the way you respond to others.

As you support learners and colleagues, you will also be influenced by their behaviour and attitude. Some PS/PA who have had particularly challenging experiences have then struggled to support learners going forward. We will look at support for the PS/PA roles later, but it is important that you consider each learner as an individual and get to know them by understanding how their experiences have shaped their knowledge, skills and behaviours.

Similarly, your learner will have previous experience. Some may have been in healthcare roles, some may have personal experiences that affect the way they behave in practice, and some may have had particularly challenging support from their PS/PA. When you looked at how you might provide induction, did you consider how you will find out about previous experiences?

Optimising the Learning Experience

We have discussed the impact of the learning environment in creating a learning culture in which everyone feels safe to make mistakes and learn from these to improve their care delivery, and you have considered some of the experiences trainees have reported in practice and reflected on your own experience. You now need to think about how you will optimise the learning experience.

It is important to bear in mind just how challenging the healthcare sector is and be realistic about how you are going to ensure that you are promoting a positive experience. Ask anyone working within the healthcare environment about their day and they will probably reflect on how busy they are, how chaotic it is trying to manage workload with significant unpredictability and the pressure they are under to meet deadlines, provide support and ensure that patient care is of a high standard. Add learners into this and the pressure increases; students report poor experiences and as a result do not want to work in the same area when qualified. For NAs, this can be your area of employment and a poor experience can result in looking for alternative work when qualified. Ensuring that students are considered part of the team around the patient will increase student satisfaction and enable the PA and PS to take opportunities to teach as they arise (the importance of effective teamwork is discussed in Chapter 7). Teachable moments are opportunities to support students to develop while continuing to manage the challenge of practice.

Teachable Moments: Creating Opportunities to Learn in Practice

Teachable moments are important in maximising the time you have to offer support and require you as a PA or PS to look for opportunities during the working day. For example, you may need to undertake a complex dressing in which the student acts predominantly as an observer but it is important to take the time before or after this to discuss why a certain dressing is being used, the expectation of wound healing and how you expect this particular patient to recover. You can consider the effect of any medication and how this impacts wound healing, the nutritional status of the patient and how as a NA this can be supported and monitored and potential plans for discharge. In these relatively short moments, you can 'bring to life' the learning that will enable the student to really understand. As a student, asking these questions and being proactive will ensure that you are an active learner rather than a passive recipient and this will help you to understand and apply this to practice going forward.

The following pointers will help you to consider teachable moments in your practice and look at creative ways to offer support (Reynolds et al. 2020).

- What teaching moments can you identify in your practice?
- How do teaching moments differ between different learners in your setting?
- What are the key skills for creating teaching moments?
- What opportunities do you have for debrief and reflection and how can they be maximised?
- How might you engage service users/patients and carers and members of the multidisciplinary team in creating and using teaching moments in practice?

As a student, you may have felt a lack of empowerment within your own learning journey which may have left you feeling that experiences offered did not reflect your needs. Consider the position asserted by the NMC and how this relates to your experiences.

> *Students should be empowered to take control of and responsibility for their own learning, and to self-direct their learning if safe and appropriate.*
>
> *(NMC 2019)*

Consider this statement in relation to your experiences and your role.

You will need to determine how you are going to translate this to your practice as you start to support others. Using teachable moments will enable you to tailor learning to the individual needs of students and give them the opportunity to establish knowledge in ways that are meaningful to their practice.

To support learners, you need to establish a 'baseline' reflecting what each individual understands about the experience they are about to undertake; this can be done formally through something like an initial interview or less formally through conversation when you first meet them. You will not always be directly responsible for assessment but you may be supervising a number of different learners and you need to understand their priorities and how they will be assessed so that you can contribute to the gathering of evidence.

As you are aware from your programme, learners may enter an environment with little if any understanding of care delivery in that setting. You have explored what makes an effective learning environment and you must ensure that the environment and support have provided the necessary guidance to enable your learner to be successful.

When you have identified what is expected of a learner, you will start to think about what level of performance you are expecting from a learner. This generally falls into three categories.

- *Skills or technique*: the way things are done, are they safe, are they adhering to policies?
- *Competence*: are they applying the theory to practice, can they explain the rationale for why things are done?
- *Professional attributes*: the approach that is taken, interpersonal relationships, behaviours and attitude.

It is important that you consider all learners in the context of what they need to know, what they have been taught so far and what their expectations are. Do not forget we are all learning all the time and at some point, you will be both the learner and 'teacher'.

Using Delegation to Support Learning

Delegation is an activity you may not have carried out within previous roles as an HCA, but as a registrant you will need to delegate and monitor the work of others (NMC 2018a). As a registrant, you need to understand your responsibility and accountability to yourself, your patients and your delegatee.

> *Delegation is the process by which you (the delegator) allocate clinical or non-clinical treatment of care to a competent person (the delegatee).*

> *You will remain responsible for the overall management of the service user, and accountable for your decision to delegate. You will not be accountable for the decisions and actions of the delegatee.*
>
> *(RCN 2024)*

The NMC states that you must be accountable for your decisions to delegate tasks and duties to other people (NMC 2018b). To achieve this, you must:

11.1 only delegate tasks and duties that are within the other person's scope of competence, making sure that they fully understand your instructions

11.2 make sure that everyone you delegate tasks to is adequately supervised and supported so they can provide safe and compassionate care

11.3 confirm that the outcome of any task you have delegated to someone else meets the required standard.

Reflective Activity

Consider, within your role as a nursing associate:

- what tasks might you delegate to others?
- what might you need to consider when delegating the task?

As a student, you are now more experienced and as you come to the end of your programme and take greater responsibility for patients, you will need to practise the art of delegation, so consider the questions above and what challenges you might face in delegating.

Barriers to Delegation

Delegation can be challenging, and it is important to understand the barriers to delegation and how you might overcome these to create a learning opportunity for yourself and others. The following are potential barriers to delegation.

- Lack of experience
- Insecurity
- Desire for control
- Lack of organisation
- Unwilling to help others develop

Magnusson et al. (2017) identified personality traits that create barriers to effective delegation.

- The do-it-all nurse – completes most of the work themselves.
- The justifier – overexplains reasons for decisions and is sometimes defensive.
- The buddy – wants to be everybody's friend and avoids assuming authority.
- The role model – hopes that others will copy their best practice but has no way of ensuring how this is done.
- The inspector – is acutely aware of their accountability and constantly checks work.

You may recognise these traits in others who have supported you but it is important to recognise them within yourself and consider how to ensure that you delegate safely and use your experience as a learning opportunity.

Delegation of a task or duty does not end at the point of delegation. The registered nurse who initiated the delegation has a duty to follow up, check that the task has been completed properly and safely, and come to a professional judgement on any measurement or assessments that have been completed (Griffith 2022).

Impact of Good Delegation

- Effective teamwork resulting in high standards of patient care.
- Provision of learning opportunities for others.
- Understanding of prior knowledge to ensure safety.
- During and after a care episode has been completed, you will be ensuring the standard has been met and providing feedback.
- Increased confidence and empowerment of the team member or learner.

When delegating any care episode, you need to ensure that the person you delegate to has the knowledge and understanding to carry out the task. You should be checking understanding and asking them to feed back to you on expectations, which will show their understanding.

If the delegated task is one that the learner is not completely confident in, you may supervise them more directly and support them through the process. You would be giving guidance and advice and referring to evidence base and policy to ensure that the standards provided match the requirements; through this, you will be teaching and supporting learning.

After any delegated episode you will provide feedback, ensuring that care has been delivered to the standard required. You might provide some reflection on what could be improved next time. You might also reflect on your own practice in terms of whether you made your instruction clear enough, and on how you determined their level of understanding.

Impact of Ineffective Delegation

We have considered the importance of delegation and how this can improve care. As an accountable practitioner, you need to understand the impact of poor or ineffective delegation.

- Missed care, including:
  - repositioning
  - mouth care
  - feeding
- Reporting observations
- Poor teamwork
- Lack of communication
- Blame culture

Providing Effective Feedback

Feedback relates to the way information is provided, in this case to the learner or student about their actions and behaviour so that they can amend practice and improve care delivery. This fosters life-long learning and improves patient care and safety. It is difficult to improve practice or services without feedback.

Reflective Activity

- Reflect on a time when you have received feedback related to your practice. How did this make you feel? Do you think this was effective in supporting you to improve practice?
- How could this have been more effective? You need to think about the impact on your future practice.

We have considered the roles of PAs and PSs in supporting students. An integral part of this support is the provision of clear and meaningful feedback which should be aimed at supporting improvement but not chastising someone for their practice. Remember that students are being supervised, so any dangerous practice should be stopped before the patient is harmed.

Feedback should support students to continue an upward spiral of performance and continual improvement. It should aim to:

- extend high-performing students
- challenge students who are coasting
- improve students who are struggling.

Through effective feedback, you should be aiming to increase students' confidence, motivation and enthusiasm for developing within their roles and provide them with insight into the standards expected in practice. Feedback should help learners to focus on specific areas and improve practice. Providing effective feedback can be difficult and whether you are giving feedback following a delegated activity or to a student who is developing their practice, you need to ensure that you have the skills to communicate effectively.

Using models for giving feedback will ensure that you remain objective and provide students with an opportunity to develop. The following is based on the Pendleton Model.

- Describe what you saw that raised your concerns. Ask if the student saw the same things.
    - Explain why this is an issue, why are you concerned.
    - Explain in more detail the implications of what happened and why it is of concern. Check that the student has insight into why this is an issue.
- Agree and commit to corrective strategies; develop a plan as to how concerns will be addressed.
    - Explore together what can be put in place to help the student correct the concern.
    - Check that the student agrees and is willing to commit to the strategy.

There is evidence that providing feedback which results in a student failing to achieve their practice requirements is so challenging that there is a culture of 'failing to fail' (Finch and Tedam 2023) which suggests that there are students who are being allowed to achieve registration but may be unfit to care for patients and therefore pose a risk to safety. It is important to understand why practice assessors and supervisors are not managing students effectively by providing feedback and making appropriate judgements. Some reasons for failing to make appropriate judgements might be:

- giving the benefit of the doubt and hoping that students will improve over time
- passing the buck, in the hope that someone else will make a judgement
- leaving it too late; it is important students are given the opportunity to amend practice or behaviours. Issues must be identified and action plans put in place to support students to develop.

To be able to address student issues and effectively provide feedback, you will need to develop resilience which has been referred to as a 'core of steel' (Hunt 2019).

Struggling Learners

Lidster and Wakefield (2022) identify the following definition in relation to students in difficulty.

> *When a student has a problem/s in their education, training, conduct or health that affects, or is likely to significantly affect, patient safety, team-working, educational progress or their own well-being.*

This definition is used widely by the medical profession but is relevant for all learners. It is important to remember that each learner has experiences both in and outside the programme and their practice experiences. You are expected to treat patients holistically so remember that the learner also needs to be considered a whole person.

When a learner is struggling for any reason, it can manifest in more errors which in turn will lead to increased frustration on the part of both learner and supervisor. This is further compounded as more people need to be involved such as academic members of staff, managers and external teams.

Learners in difficulty may be able to demonstrate the skills required for practice outcomes but may not meet professional expectations in terms of conduct and behaviour and may not display the appropriate attitude. Learners who are struggling may exhibit a range of behaviours.

- Emotional responses
  - Anger
  - Fear
  - Hostility
  - Disappointment

- ▨ Behavioural responses
  - ▨ Rudeness
  - ▨ Impatience
  - ▨ Avoidance
- ▨ Manifestations of poorly performing learners
  - ▨ Appear uninterested
  - ▨ Lack motivation
  - ▨ Time keeping: late to work, taking extended breaks
  - ▨ Poor interpersonal relationships with patients/carers/MDT
  - ▨ Not adhering to uniform policy

When faced with a student who is struggling, you need to utilise all the skills you have learnt around identifying concerns, feeding back appropriately and providing the student with clear direction as to how to improve. You will need to discuss attitudes and behaviours as well as skills and practical development and be able to provide them with guidance as to how to improve. Where students fail to meet the standards expected, you may need to make challenging decisions and potentially fail students.

The challenges of supporting learners are increasing as there are more students in practice from a broader range of different programmes. Recruitment to healthcare roles is not meeting the demand of services so the number of students is increasing, placing increased pressure on placements.

While you will be recognised as a PS when you have registered with the NMC, you need to consolidate your practice and should be supported when you are supporting others. During or after preceptorship, you will be able to complete some additional training to become a PA when you will look in more detail at the evidence needed to complete the final assessment of a period of learning. As a PS, you will contribute to this evidence.

Chapter Summary

This chapter has explored the complexities of supporting students in the practice setting and has considered your transition from student to supervisor or assessor. Practice learning is multifaceted and you will develop skills as you progress through preceptorship and as you grow in confidence. There are many ways in which learners can be supported creatively. You need to look at your own experience and ensure that you are working with your learner to establish ways of support and assessment which enable your learner to evidence their skills and abilities.

References

Dainty, A.D., Barnes, D., Bellamy, E. et al. (2021). Opportunity, support and understanding: the experience of four early trainee nursing associates. *British Journal of Healthcare Assistants* 15 (6): 284–291.

Department of Health and Social Care and Independent Maternity Review (2022). *Findings, Conclusions and Essential Actions from the Independent Review of Maternity Services at the Shrewsbury and Telford Hospital NHS Trust: Ockenden Report – Final*. London: Stationery Office.

Duffy, K. and Gillies, A. (2018). Supervision and assessment: the new nursing and midwifery council standards. *Nursing Management* 25 (3): 17–21.

Finch, J. and Tedam, P. (2023). Failure to fail or fast tracking to failure: a critical exploration of social work placements. *Social Work Education* 43 (7): 2024–2039.

Francis, R. (2013). *Report of the Mid Staffordshire NHS Foundation Trust Public Inquiry – Executive Summary*. London: HMSO.

Griffith, R. (2022). The nurse's legal duty to safely delegate tasks and to follow up the outcome. *British Journal of Nursing* 31 (7): 400–401.

Henderson, A. and Eaton, E. (2013). Assisting nurses to facilitate student and new graduate learning in practice settings: what "support" do nurses at the bedside need? *Nurse Education in Practice* 13 (3): 197–201.

Henderson, A., Briggs, J., Schoonbeek, S., and Paterson, K. (2011). A framework to develop a clinical learning culture in health facilities: ideas from the literature. *International Nursing Review* 58 (2): 196–202.

Hunt, L.A. (2019). Developing a "core of steel": the key attributes of effective practice assessors. *British Journal of Nursing* 28 (22): 1478–1484.

King, R., Ryan, T., Wood, E. et al. (2020). Motivations, experiences and aspirations of trainee nursing associates in England: a qualitative study. *BMC Health Services Research* 20 (1): 802.

Levett-Jones, T., Lathlean, J., Higgins, I., and McMillan, M. (2009). Staff–student relationships and their impact on nursing students' belongingness and learning. *Journal of Advanced Nursing* 65 (2): 316–324.

Lidster, J. and Wakefield, S. (2022). *Student Practice Supervision and Assessment*, 2e. London: Sage.

Magnusson, C., Allan, H., Horton, K. et al. (2017). An analysis of delegation styles among newly qualified nurses. *Nursing Standard* 31 (25): 46–53.

Nursing and Midwifery Council (NMC) (2018a). *Future Nurse: Standards of Proficiency for Registered Nurses*. London: Nursing and Midwifery Council.

Nursing and Midwifery Council (NMC) (2018b). *Standards Framework for Nursing and Midwifery Education*. London: Nursing and Midwifery Council.

Nursing and Midwifery Council (NMC) (2018c). *Standards of Proficiency for Nursing Associates*. London: Nursing and Midwifery Council.

Nursing and Midwifery Council (NMC) (2019). The student at the centre of learning. www.nmc.org.uk/supporting-information-on-standards-for-student-supervision-and-assessment-old/student-empowerment/the-student-at-the-centre-of-learning/#:~:text=Students%20should%20be%20empowered%20to,independent%2C%20reflective%20and%20professional%20practitioners

Reynolds, L.M., Attenborough, J., and Halse, J. (2020). Nurses as educators: creating teachable moments in practice. *Nursing Times* 116 (2): 25–28.

Royal College of Nursing (RCN) (2024). Accountability and delegation guide. www.rcn.org.uk/Professional-Development/Accountability-and-delegation/Guide

Vanson, T. and Beckett, A. (2018). *Evaluation of the Introduction of the Nursing Associate*, 50. London: Traverse.

Further Reading

Nursing and Midwifery Council (NMC) (2018). *The Code. Professional Standards of Practice and Behaviour for Nurses, Midwives and Nursing Associates*. London: Nursing and Midwifery Council.

Index

Page number followed by 'f' refers to figures. Page numbers followed by 't' refer to tables.

The Nursing Associate: Stepping into Practice, First Edition. Edited by Annabel Coulson.
© 2025 John Wiley & Sons Ltd. Published 2025 by John Wiley & Sons Ltd.